ESTROGEN REPLACEMENT THERAPY

by

R. Don Gambrell, Jr., M.D.

Clinical Professor
Department of Obstetrics and Gynecology
and Physiology and Endocrinology
Medical College of Georgia
Augusta, GA 30912-3395

2nd Edition

Essential
Information Systems, Inc.
P.O. Box 811247
Dallas, TX 75381

For Direct Mail Orders, Write:

Essential Medical Information Systems, Inc.
P.O. Box 811247
Dallas, TX 75381

For Phone Orders, Call:

1-800-225-0694

ISBN: 0-929240-09-X

SECOND EDITION

Published in the United States 1990

Center Index Texts Published by
Essential Medical Information Systems, Inc.:

Request Catalog for complete list of center index texts.

Table of Contents

Tables

Figures

CENTER INDEX SYSTEM

The purpose of the center index system is to enable readers to immediately locate all the information contained in the book. Tabs are provided with each center index so there is a direct connection between the center index and text. The text is organized in a sequential format to enable the reader to proceed to any area of the text without having to read through information not relevant to the situation.

Dedication

This book is dedicated to my wife, Caroline, who for more than 30 years has supported my every endeavor with love, warmth and kind understanding.

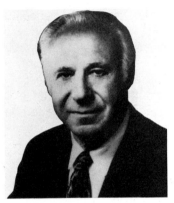

Robert B. Greenblatt, M.D.
1906-1987

This book is also dedicated to the memory of Dr. Robert B. Greenblatt, my mentor and colleague, who for 19 years continued to teach me scientific discipline, diligence and compassion. His dedication to the betterment of women, particularly their hormone problems and especially the menopause, has greatly improved their quality of life. This book is an extension of Dr. Greenblatt's work, who first advocated safe hormone replacement in 1945, by adding cyclic progestogens to shed the endometrium in estrogen-treated women. His memory will live on as the many physicians he trained and stimulated continue the work he started more than 50 years ago.

#1 Introduction

Menopausal Hormone Deficiency

After the menopause, the average woman still has one-third of her lifespan ahead. However, women's experience of the menopause and its effects on their remaining years vary widely.

The declining ovarian function can be rapid for some and slower for others. Some women produce sufficient endogenous estrogens to remain asymptomatic, but others develop a variety of disturbances during the climacteric — a term in current use for the premenopausal, menopausal and postmenopausal period.

These symptoms may include:

- Hot flushes (or flashes)
- Night sweats
- Vaginal irritation or dryness
- Insomnia
- Depression

The issue of what should be done about adverse climacteric symptoms is controversial. There is general agreement that menopause is a hormone-deficient state. The disagreement arises over whether the hormone deficiency should be treated and to what degree.

Some physicians believe that the menopause is a physiologic event and that any attempt to correct estrogen deficiency is an intrusion into the natural aging process. Some contend that menopausal symptoms are psychoneurotic. Others contend that only vasomotor manifestations (hot flushes, sweats) and atrophic vaginitis are directly due to the estrogen deficit, and that these manifestations may be treated with the smallest possible dose of oral estrogens for a short period of time.

Trends in Treatment

Estrogen replacement therapy is controversial. It was fashionable in the 1960s, but in the 1970s complications became apparent. Physicians became reluctant to treat the climacteric and patients became wary of hormone therapy because of widely publicized reports that estrogens caused endometrial cancer. In the 1980s, however, hormone therapy is once again growing in popularity.

First, there has been a recently-growing recognition of the dangers of long-term estrogen deficiency. This deficiency can lead to development of:

- Osteoporosis
- Atherosclerotic heart disease
- Possible psychogenic manifestations

There is growing acknowledgement that estrogen deficiency should be treated as vigorously as any other endocrinopathy and without a necessary limitation of time. Instead of the minimal treatments suggested in the past to alleviate specific symptoms, some women require hormonal therapy for years instead of months, continuously instead of cyclically and in larger dosages than previously recommended. Further, there is a recognition that some postmenopausal women need treatment with other hormones, such as progestogen, to prevent endometrial hyperplasia and subsequent neoplasia.

Second, the belief that estrogen treatment causes endometrial cancer is no longer valid. The incidence of cancer of the endometrium or of the breast need not increase as a result of long-term estrogen therapy if cyclic progestogens in adequate dosages are added to the estrogen regimen.

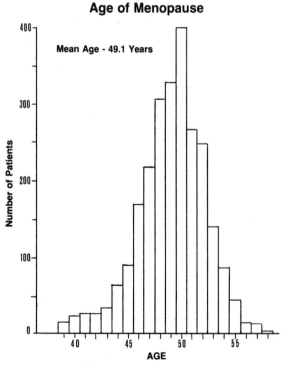

FIGURE 1. The age of menopause in over 2,000 women undergoing a natural menopause (Reproduced with permission of the publisher, the American Fertility Society, from Gambrell) (Ref 25).

Notes

#2 Vasomotor Symptoms

2. Clinical Information

Most women who seek medical attention for menopausal symptoms complain of vasomotor symptoms. These include:

- Hot flushes (or flashes)
- Night sweats

These symptoms usually have an insidious onset and increase as serum estrogens decline. Vasomotor symptoms are variable in frequency and severity and may persist for several months to a few years.

Research

Studies have shown an association between the pulsatile release of LH and the occurrence of hot flushes. However, LH levels per se are not responsible for triggering vasomotor symptoms, since these phenomena can occur after hypophysectomy. If untreated, the hypothalamus and autonomic nervous systems gradually adjust to the lower levels of estrogen and eventually hot flushes will abate.

Patients with gonadal dysgenesis have high levels of gonadotrophins; however, these individuals experience vasomotor symptoms only after exposure to exogenous estrogens and subsequent withdrawal.

Recommendations

In the past, low dosages of estrogen have been given for short intervals and then reduced gradually so that hot flushes fade. This concept is no longer valid. A woman experiencing menopausal symptoms has become estrogen-deficient and will remain so for the rest of her life.

A balanced program of estrogen replacement therapy combined with cyclic progestogens is the best treatment, since the real goal of estrogen replacement is not only to alleviate vasomotor symptoms but to prevent later metabolic consequences such as osteoporosis and atherosclerosis.

#3 Urogenital Atrophy

Clinical Information

3. Atrophy of the genital epithelium may result in senile vaginitis (Ref 7). Symptoms may include:

- Irritation
- Burning
- Pruritis
- Leukorrhea
- Dyspareunia
- Vaginal bleeding
- Decrease of vaginal secretions
- Thinning and easily-traumatized epithelium
- Shortening and lessening of distensibility of the vagina

Most sexual problems experienced by post-menopausal women are due to the physical status of the vaginal mucosa, which must maintain sufficient protective moisture and provide lubrication during coitus. After menopause, atrophic changes may lead to:

- Dyspareunia
- Vaginitis
- Vaginismus
- Physical discomfort
- Loss of sexual interest

Research

Studies have demonstrated (Ref 72) that the estrogen-deprived state in postmenopausal women leads to changes in:

- Quantity of vaginal fluid
- pH levels
- Vaginal blood flow

However, urogenital changes which develop because of estrogen deprivation are reversible with estrogen replacement therapy, although the longer the estrogen deprivation, the slower the physiologic response.

Recommendations

The preferred treatment for atrophic vaginitis is local estrogen therapy in the form of vaginal creams (such as Premarin and Estrace), which are well absorbed into the vaginal mucosa. Daily h.s. applications should be given for 1 to 2 weeks, then 3 times a week thereafter is normally sufficient for maintenance (see Section #13).

Systemic therapy by oral or other routes is usually started simultaneously. Local vaginal therapy can sometimes be discontinued after a few months, or continued vaginal cream treatment may be required in addition to systemic estrogens. Irritative symptoms abate rapidly with estrogen vaginal cream but restoration of normal vaginal blood flow may take up to a year.

To a lesser extent, the vulvar epithelium also becomes thin and may be irritated or subject to infection. These conditions commonly respond to applications of vaginal estrogen cream, but a 1% or 2% testosterone cream may be necessary for kaurosis vulva or other atrophic or leukoplakic vulvar conditions. Vulvar pruritis may sometimes require 1% hydrocortisone creams or other glucocorticoid creams for relief in addition to either estrogen or testosterone creams.

The integrity of the lower urinary tract mucosa is dependent upon estrogens. Estrogen deficiency may therefore result in irritative symptoms such as:

- Dysuria
- Burning on urination
- Cystitis
- Urethral caruncles
- Non-gonococcal urethritis

These respond best to local applications of vaginal estrogen creams with the simultaneous initiation of oral estrogen therapy.

Notes

#4 Psychogenic Manifestations

Clinical Information

Many postmenopausal women complain of psychogenic disturbances. These may include:

- Increased nervousness
- Depression
- Anxiety
- Insomnia
- Headaches

Other conditions that may be aggravated by menopausal symptoms include:

- Preexisting psychosomatic problems intensified by hot flushes
- Sleep patterns disturbed by night sweats
- Libido decreased due to atrophic vaginitis resulting in dyspareunia

Research

Carefully controlled double-blind and cross-over studies indicate that estrogens have a tonic mental effect (Ref 25). Patients had higher scores on psychometric evaluation (Ref 87), alleviating the psychogenic manifestations independent of vasomotor symptoms (Ref 11).

Moderate to severe depression, as measured by the Zung Self-Rating Depression Scale, was significantly higher in patients who had a surgical menopause by hysterectomy with or without bilateral oophorectomy, when compared to women undergoing a natural menopause (Ref 2). This suggests that women undergoing pelvic surgery have either not been reconciled to its necessity or were insufficiently prepared for its consequences.

In a study using pellets of estradiol, testosterone or a placebo, testosterone increased the frequency and intensity of orgasmic responses (Ref 80). In a double-blind study using hot flushes as the main index, 96% of patients improved on estrogens and 91% on an estrogen-androgen combination. Fair to good results were obtained in 56% of patients receiving androgens and 16% of those given a placebo. The estrogen-androgen combination was associated with less withdrawal bleeding and accentuated well-being and libido (Ref 78).

Headaches in postmenopausal women are frequently regarded as psychosomatic and not hormone-related, but in one study using estrogen, progestogen and placebo, headaches were alleviated while high levels of estrogen were maintained (Ref 21).

In a study of 85 patients receiving hormone replacement therapy when headaches were a secondary complaint, relief from headaches was obtained by the administration of estradiol pellets alone or in combination with testosterone (Ref 39).

Although these studies may not prove that psychogenic complaints of postmenopausal women are hormone-dependent, they indicate that many are hormone-responsive, since patients improve once therapy is begun.

Recommendations

Sexual dysfunction in the menopausal woman, long regarded by psychologists and sex therapists as psychogenic, has been shown to be responsive to hormone therapy. Relief may be afforded by estrogens, including estrogen vaginal cream, for complaints such as vaginal dryness and dyspareunia and by androgens for complaints of loss of sexual interest (see Section #14).

It is important to note that a postmenopausal woman who has lost up to two-thirds of estrogen production has also lost up to one-half of androgen production. Although most postmenopausal women respond well to estrogen-progestogen therapy, some require the addition of an androgen. Women treated with estrogen-androgen replacement therapy were more composed, elated and energetic than those treated with estrogen alone (Ref 74). The addition of androgen did enhance sexual desire and increased the frequency of sexual fantasies when compared to estrogen alone or with placebo. In the Yale Mid-Life Study Program, androgens are not routinely prescribed unless there is a deficiency in the total or free testosterone levels (Ref 71).

Notes

#5 Osteoporosis

Clinical Information

Osteoporosis is a skeletal disorder primarily affecting trabecular bone in which a reduction in the quantity of bone predisposes to fracture. Although both sexes lose bone mass with aging, it is rare for men to develop symptomatic osteoporosis before age 70.

This is a major public health problem affecting 20,000,000 older Americans of which 90% are postmenopausal women (Ref 65). It has been estimated that there are 1,700,000 fractures each year due to osteoporosis, at an annual public health cost in excess of $3.8 billion. Approximately 25% of white women over the age of 60 have spinal compression fractures. This number increases to 50% by the age of 75. With increasing longevity, a woman reaching the age of 50 now has a life expectancy of 80.4 years, when the already serious morbidity and mortality associated with postmenopausal osteoporosis becomes even greater. Of all hip fractures, 80% are associated with osteoporosis and 34% of all elderly patients with hip fractures die within 6 months (Ref 38).

Research

Several studies have been conducted into the effects of estrogen therapy on the prevention of osteoporosis. These studies have demonstrated that estrogen therapy:

- Prevents osteoporosis

- Decreases vertebral, hip and other fractures
- Prevents further loss of height

In one long-term prospective study of 1,000 women treated with estrogens for 15 years (14,318 patient-years of observation), wrist fractures were reduced by 70% from the expected rate (Ref 8). No hip fractures occurred during 15 years of estrogen therapy in these 1,000 women. In a carefully controlled ongoing study from the Mayo Clinic, patients treated with calcium carbonate, 1,500 to 2,000 mg daily, had 419 fractures per 1,000 patient-years of observation compared to 834 per 1,000 in the placebo-treated group (Ref 67). Fracture rate was reduced by 61% to 304 per 1,000 in those treated with calcium plus sodium fluoride, 50 to 60 mg daily.

However, the most effective therapy, with a fracture rate of 53 per 1,000, was the combination of:

- Conjugated estrogens, 0.625 to 2.5 mg daily
- Sodium fluoride
- Calcium

The addition of vitamin D had no significant effect and was associated with a substantial incidence of hypercalcemia or hypercalciuria. Thus, the Mayo group did not believe that vitamin D should be included in therapy for osteoporosis.

Recommendations

The recommendations of the National Institutes of Health Consensus Development Conference on Osteoporosis are:

- That estrogen therapy is the best prevention and treatment of osteoporosis
- That calcium supplementation, which should be begun about age 40 or approximately 10 years prior to menopause, should be given in dosages of 1,000 mg of elemental calcium daily (see Section #16)
- That weight-bearing exercise is the best activity to prevent osteoporosis (Ref 65)

An international consensus conference confirmed that estrogen replacement, supplemental calcium and exercise were the mainstays in prevention of osteoporosis (Ref 3). Fluoride may increase trabecular bone mass but should not be used in predominantly cortical osteoporosis nor does it have a place in the prophylaxis of bone loss. Vitamin D and anabolic steroids do not have a place in preventing osteoporosis. Calcitonin may be useful in women at high risk where estrogens are contraindicated (see Section #26). Cyclic and coherence therapies (ADFR) are promising but need more research.

Conjugated estrogens, 0.625 mg daily, is the dosage of estrogen shown to prevent osteoporosis in 90% of postmenopausal women. Higher dosages of estrogen, such as 1.25 to 2.5 mg, are required if osteoporosis is already present (Ref 22, 55).

An injectable progestogen may also be added to help prevent bone loss.

Prevention

Prevention of postmenopausal osteoporosis may not be unique to estrogens, since therapy with an injectable progestogen is also effective in preventing bone loss (Ref 54). The addition of a progestogen to estrogen therapy may be important in preventing osteoporosis but may be essential in treating patients who already have osteoporosis (Ref 84).

While most studies indicate that estrogen therapy inhibits the resorption of calcium from bone, most likely by restoring calcitonin levels that are decreased after menopause, at least 3 studies have shown that combination estrogen-progestogen therapy may actually increase bone mass by promoting new bone formation.

In a 10-year double-blind prospective study, significant differences were observed between patients receiving cyclic estrogen-progestogen therapy and a group given placebo (Ref 59). In women given combination estrogen-progestogen therapy less than 3 years after the onset of menopause, bone density actually increased. Although there was some bone demineralization in the estrogen-progestogen users when therapy was started later than 3 years after menopause, the loss of bone mass was significantly less than in either placebo group. This study emphasizes the importance of beginning estrogen-progestogen replacement early into menopause, but it also indicates that these hormones are beneficial to osteoporotic women, regardless of age. It should be noted that conjugated estrogens, 2.5 mg daily, was the dosage used in this study.

In a crossover study comparing the effects of estrogen-progestogen therapy with placebo, bone mineral content increased during the 3 years of combination hormone therapy but continued to decline in the placebo-treated group (Ref 14).

When some patients in the estrogen-progestogen group were changed to placebo, bone density decreased. Bone mass also increased in placebo-treated women after being changed to active hormone therapy.

Another group (Ref 19) compared the effects of estrogen only to estrogen-progestogen combination on the metabolic parameters of bone loss:

- Plasma calcium
- Urinary calcium/creatinine ratio
- Hydroxyproline

All values were diminished with estrogen therapy and decreased further when a progestogen was added to the estrogen.

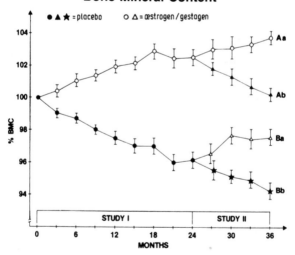

Bone Mineral Content

FIGURE 2. Bone mineral content as a function of time and treatment in postmenopausal women (Reproduced with permission of the author and publisher) (Ref 14).

Notes

#6 Coronary Artery Disease

Clinical Information

Myocardial infarction rarely occurs in women prior to menopause. Younger women who have had bilateral oophorectomy demonstrate a higher incidence of myocardial infarction unless estrogen replacement is begun soon after the ovaries are removed. The greatest benefit that will accrue to postmenopausal estrogen users is prevention of coronary artery disease. Over 400,000 women die every year in the U.S. from heart attacks.

6. Research

Estrogen therapy for prevention of coronary artery disease fell into disrepute over a decade ago when men with prior myocardial infarction were treated with high dosages of estrogen in an effort to reduce the risk of recurrent infarction (Ref 15). Men given 5 mg of conjugated estrogens daily experienced twice the number of nonfatal myocardial infarctions, 3 times the number of pulmonary emboli, and 1.5 times the number of deaths as did the placebo group.

In addition, retrospective studies linked oral contraceptives to heart disease in relatively young women, with the number suffering myocardial infarction invariably higher among those who smoked. The latest Royal College of General Practitioners' study does not show any excess deaths from heart disease in users of the new low-dosage birth control pills except in those beyond the age of 45 who also smoke (Ref 51).

Prevention

Several recent studies suggest that estrogens may exert a protective effect against cardiovascular disease, especially when the low dosages of natural estrogens sufficient to relieve menopausal symptoms are used. A 63% decrease in expected deaths from heart disease was observed in 1,000 estrogen-treated women followed for 15 years (Ref 8).

In estrogen-treated women followed up to 25 years and compared to those never taking estrogens (Ref 42), a significant decrease was found in:

- Coronary artery disease
- Congestive heart failure
- Atherosclerotic cardiovascular disease
- Hypertension

The Nurses' Health Study (Ref 77) confirmed that:

- Postmenopausal estrogen use significantly reduced the risk of coronary disease (RR = 0.5; P = 0.007)
- Current use reduced the risk even lower (RR = 0.3; P = 0.001)
- These benefits held after adjustment for factors such as:
  - Smoking
  - Hypertension
  - Diabetes
  - High cholesterol
  - Parental history of myocardial infarctions
  - Past use of oral contraceptives
  - Obesity

In a cohort of 2,270 women from The Lipid Research Clinics followed for eight years, there were 44 deaths due to cardiovascular disease among 1,677 nonusers and six deaths in the 593 estrogen users (RR=0.34) (Ref 9). This study concluded that the protective effect of estrogen is mediated through increased HDL levels.

An epidemiologic study indicated a significant reduction in the death rate of acute myocardial infarction among users of estrogen (RR = 0.59, P = 0.002) (Ref 45). A reduced hospitalization rate for coronary artery disease was also observed for estrogen users compared to nonusers.

Almost every other study has confirmed the protective effect of estrogen use upon coronary atherosclerosis even after adjustment for age, cigarette smoking, diabetes, cholesterol and hypertension (Ref 40, 82). Higher HDL levels among estrogen users may indicate the biologic mechanism by which postmenopausal estrogen use lowers the risk of coronary occlusion. Only one study failed to confirm the beneficial effect of estrogens upon heart disease. The Framingham Heart Study (Ref 91) confirmed significant improvement in estrogen users when compared with nonusers in:

- HDL cholesterol
- Low density lipoprotein (LDL)
- Total cholesterol to HDL cholesterol ratio

This study concluded that estrogen use produced a more favorable lipid pattern, but that cardiovascular mortality did not differ between estrogen users and the controls.

Notes

#7 Vaginal Hormonal Cytology

Clinical Information

A patient's complaints of menopausal symptoms may be sufficient reason to begin estrogen replacement therapy (see Section #1). However, the vaginal smear is a good reflection of endogenous estrogen production.

With normal endogenous estrogen, there should be a high percentage (15-30%) of superficial cells (cells with small pyknotic nuclei and a large amount of cytoplasm) and the remaining cells should be of the intermediate types (larger nuclei with the nucleolus visible but still mostly cytoplasm). When parabasal cells (with a nucleus-to-cytoplasmic ratio of 50:50 or greater) are present on the vaginal smear, the patient usually has decreased estrogen production. If the vaginal smear is comprised of more than 50% parabasal cells, the patient is in a very hypoestrogenic state.

The physician can prepare the smear and read the vaginal hormonal cytology himself, providing instant information, or send the vaginal smear to a cytology or pathology lab for a report of the maturation index report (the percentage of superficial, intermediate, and parabasal cells). Most Pap smear reports now list an estrogen index.

Cytology Procedure

The smear is best taken from the lateral vaginal wall because it is usually more free of mucus and debris. A good instant stain for vaginal hormonal cytology is 1% pinacyanol. The pinacyanol chloride powder dye is obtained from the

Eastman Kodak Company and the solution is made with one gram of dye in 100 cc of 90-95% alcohol, either ethanol or methanol.

After smearing the vaginal mucosa cells on a glass slide, a few drops of pinacyanol are applied, allowed to dry for one minute, then rinsed with ordinary tap water. Slides are long-lasting and the purple color can be freshened with drops of water or oil.

Fern Pattern Procedure

Another simple test used for estimation of estrogen production is the fern pattern of cervical mucus, although this can only be used in patients who have not had a hysterectomy.

Mucus from the cervix is smeared onto a glass slide and allowed to dry for 5 minutes. If the fern pattern appears under the microscope, normal estrogen production is indicated, since the salts only crystallize with estrogen unopposed by progesterone.

During the normal ovulatory cycle, the fern pattern of cervical mucus increases from menses until ovulation, and then rapidly disappears after ovulation due to progesterone. The fern pattern is also absent during pregnancy even though estrogen levels are high, because the high progesterone levels keep the cervical mucus from ferning.

Summary

Vaginal hormonal cytology and cervical mucus fern pattern cannot be used to diagnose menopause nor to follow the effects of estrogen therapy, but these are adjunctive simple methods useful in evaluation of patients with menopausal symptoms.

Estrogen replacement therapy should not be denied to severely symptomatic women on the basis of what appears to be a normal estrogen smear. Consideration should also be given to initiating hormone replacement in asymptomatic postmenopausal women with very hypoestrogenic vaginal smears. The latter group would possibly benefit from additional testing for osteoporosis risk by dual photon absorptiometry.

Most symptomatic postmenopausal women need no additional testing other than the simple measures outlined above and the basic routine tests (see Section #11).

Notes

#8 Progestogen Challenge Test

Clinical Information

The progestogen challenge test should be administered to all postmenopausal women with an intact uterus at annual evaluation. Included are:

- Symptomatic women being evaluated for estrogen replacement therapy
- Estrogen-treated patients not already on progestogen therapy
- Asymptomatic postmenopausal women

It is the most reliable test for assessing potential estrogenic stimulation of the endometrium.

Not all postmenopausal women need estrogen replacement therapy, since many produce sufficient endogenous estrogens to remain asymptomatic and prevent the metabolic changes of estrogen deficiency in later life, such as atrophic vaginitis, osteoporosis and atherosclerosis. However, within this group may be those in greatest need of cyclic progestogen therapy to prevent endometrial hyperplasia, which may lead to adenocarcinoma.

Research

The progestogen challenge test was a concept evolved at Wilford Hall USAF Medical Center when it was recognized that the second highest incidence of endometrial cancer was observed in untreated postmenopausal women (Ref 28, 31).

Original work on the progestogen challenge test has been confirmed by a prospective study utilizing 100 mg of progesterone in oil given in-tramuscularly (Ref 44). In a study of 30 asymp-tomatic postmenopausal women, five had with-drawal bleeding to the progestogen challenge, and three of these five (60%) had either adenomatous or atypical adenomatous hyperpla-sia. In the 25 subjects with no withdrawal bleeding the endometrial histology was normal, mostly atrophic or inactive endometrium. There were no adenocarcinomas in either group, and although the number of subjects was small, the difference between the two groups was statistically signifi-cant ($P \leq 0.001$).

In the second phase of this study, in which 10 patients with known adenomatous hyperplasia were tested, the progestogen challenge resulted in withdrawal bleeding in 9 (90%), confirming the effectiveness of this test in detecting abnormal endometrial pathology.

The conclusion was that the progestogen challenge test was a reliable screening test for detecting women at greater risk for developing endometrial hyperplasia or adenocarcinoma.

Procedure

The progestogen challenge test is performed by administering a 13-day course of progestogen, either Provera 10 mg or Aygestin 5 mg, to all postmenopausal women with an intact uterus (see Section #15).

If a positive response occurs, as manifested by withdrawal bleeding, progestogen should be continued for 13 days each month for as long as withdrawal bleeding follows. If there is a negative response, it is recommended that the progestogen challenge be repeated each year for asymptomatic postmenopausal women not using any hormones. Annual endometrial biopsies are not necessary in estrogen-progestogen users (see Section #9). Because of the benefits of added progestogen upon the bones and the breast (see Section #5 and #19), this hormone should be continued in estrogen users, whether they are having withdrawal bleeding or not.

Notes

#9 Endometrial Biopsy

Clinical Information

Women receiving unopposed estrogen therapy should have annual endometrial biopsies. Postmenopausal women with any abnormal bleeding should have one of the following:

- An extensive endometrial biopsy
- Clinic curettage
- Formal D & C

Perimenopausal women who have irregular menses should have each of the following:

- An extensive endometrial sampling
- Pap smear
- Cervical biopsy, after Schiller's stain or colposcopically-directed
- Endocervical curettage
- Bimanual examination

An exception to the above in estrogen-progestogen users is when bleeding occurs on or after day eleven of progestogen therapy, no evaluation is necessary since the histology has been shown to be predominantly secretory (Ref 63).

Endometrial Evaluation Methods

The traditional method for evaluating the endometrium has been diagnostic dilatation and curettage (D & C). However, hospitalization for a D & C, even on an outpatient basis, has disadvantages, including:

- Increased anesthetic risk
- Additional expense
- Delay in diagnosis

These problems can be avoided by a properly-performed clinic or office curettage, performed by carefully utilizing the Randall or Novak endometrial suction biopsy with 12 to 16 strokes. The endometrial cavity should be sampled twice when minimal tissue is obtained, and 3 times or more if much tissue is extracted. This process will yield as much information as a hospital D & C.

Although there is patient discomfort with this office procedure, it may be minimized by gentleness and a careful explanation of each step. Discomfort can also be reduced by placing 4% Zylocaine on a small cotton-tipped applicator in the endocervical canal for 3 to 5 minutes. Paracervical blocks can also be performed; however, these may be more painful than the procedure itself.

Other satisfactory endometrial evaluation methods include:

- Curity Isaacs Endometrial Cell Sampler
- The Vabra Aspirator
- The Milex Endometrial Cannula
- Unimar Pipelle Endometrial Suction Curette

Summary

Endometrial biopsies are desirable before beginning estrogen replacement therapy, but may only be necessary for those who respond by bleeding in the progestogen challenge test (see Section #8).

Progestogen challenge tests were not performed in the Wilford Hall USAF Medical Center studies (Ref 31, 36). Consequently, most of the endometrial cancers in the estrogen-progestogen users were probably already present from the unopposed estrogens before the progestogen was added. If the progestogen challenge test is utilized as directed, patients with a negative response (no withdrawal bleeding) do not need an endometrial biopsy.

In addition, it is easier to perform the biopsy if the patient returns on the first or second day of withdrawal bleeding. In approximately 10 to 15% of postmenopausal women, the cervix is so stenotic that endometrial biopsies are difficult to perform in the office. Withdrawal bleeding dilates the cervix slightly, which facilitates sounding and performance of the biopsy in the clinic.

Notes

#10 Osteoporosis Detection Methods

Types of Methods Available

There are at least three methods of screening women to find which patients are losing bone. These methods of determining bone mass include:

- Regular x-rays
- Single and dual photon absorptiometry
- Quantitative CAT-scan

Regular X-Rays

Regular x-rays of the bones can reveal osteoporosis. However, before osteoporosis can be detected on regular x-rays, a person has to lose 30% to 40% of total bone mass. This is a fairly late stage of the disease.

Newer and better methods will reveal lesser amounts of bone loss to allow earlier detection and prompt treatment of the condition.

Single and Dual Photon Absorptiometry

10.

Photon absorptiometry is a new technique that will detect small amounts of bone loss, allowing diagnosis and treatment of osteoporosis much sooner than x-rays. Other advantages are very low radiation exposure, about 1/100 that of standard x-rays.

Single photon absorptiometry is used to measure bone mass in the radius using radioactive iodine (I-131). The amount of radiation that passes through the bone is measured by a detector positioned above the arm, thus determining the thickness of the bone.

Dual photon absorptiometry uses radioactive gadolinium (Gd-153) as the radiation source. It is used to measure bone thickness in the vertebrae and in the hip. A dual beam of Gd-153 is passed through the spine or hip and the amount of radiation that passes through is measured by a detector positioned above the body, registering the thickness of the bone.

With both single and dual photon absorptiometry, computers are used to determine the percent of bone present, compared with standard amounts of bone found in women the same age and normal amounts in young women. These standards of bone mass that should be present were worked out at the University of Wisconsin. The report printed out by the computer informs the physician about bone mass information which includes:

- The patient's bone thickness
- How it compares to others of her age
- How much bone mass has been lost since menopause

The report also indicates, in a graph, whether the degree of the patient's risk for fracture is:

- Normal
- Mild
- Moderate
- Severe

Quantitative Computed Axial Tomography (CAT)

A CAT scan is the most accurate measurement of bone but it is relatively expensive. Also, since it uses x-rays as the radiation source, the amount of radiation exposure is considerably higher than with dual radiation absorptiometry (13 to 20 times higher).

In young women whose ovaries have been removed, a CAT scan can detect bone loss in the spine very early, as soon as two to four months after the operation (Ref 22). It is, therefore, very useful in research on osteoporosis but is not necessary in evaluating patients for estrogen therapy.

Need for Bone Measurements

Most women do not need any of these osteoporosis screening methods, but for medical researchers these tests are essential to determine:

- Dosages of estrogen
- Need for supplemental calcium
- Addition of other therapies:
  - Vitamin D
  - Progestogens
  - Sodium fluoride

These tests may also be useful in following patients who already have osteoporosis to ensure that the progression of osteoporosis has been stopped with the present therapy.

If patients will seek medical evaluation for estrogen deficiency and physicians will treat patients for estrogen deficiency, osteoporosis can be prevented.

It is known that oral therapy with 0.625 mg of conjugated estrogens will prevent osteoporosis in over 90% of postmenopausal women. There is very active clinical research being conducted on other types of estrogens to determine the dosages necessary to prevent osteoporosis.

Osteoporosis Screening Clinics

A number of osteoporosis screening clinics are springing up across the United States, and they are beneficial since they are increasing the public awareness of osteoporosis. Most of these use the single and dual photon absorptiometry methods of screening.

However, most women do not need to be screened for osteoporosis. They only need to be treated with estrogens if they are estrogen-deficient. It is far better to prevent bone loss than it is to treat osteoporosis.

Who Should Be Screened?

There are certain known factors that increase the risk for osteoporosis (Ref 54). It is not unreasonable to screen women who have multiple risk factors including:

- White or Asian heritage
- A positive family history of osteoporosis
- Low calcium intake (lifelong)
- Early menopause

- Ovaries removed at a young age
- Sedentary lifestyle
- No children
- Alcohol abuse
- High salt intake
- Cigarette smoking
- High caffeine intake
- High protein intake
- High phosphate intake
- Diseases such as hyperthyroidism
- Certain drugs such as steroids

Notes

#11 Laboratory and Other Tests

Basic Tests

There are a number of basic tests that should be performed when evaluating a patient for estrogen replacement therapy. These include:

- Blood pressure
- Electrolytes
- Liver function
- Renal function
- Enzymes
- CBC
- Blood indices
- Platelet count
- Thyroxine
- Urinalysis

Additional tests should be obtained if indicated from the history. For example, with a past history of nontraumatic thromboembolic disease, then the following should be added to the platelet count:

- Prothrombin time
- Partial thromboplastin time
- Antithrombin III

11.

Consideration should be given to fractionization of cholesterol into HDL, LDL and VLDL, since HDL cholesterol may be decreased after menopause.

These routine tests should be repeated after 6 months of estrogen therapy and repeated approximately every 2 years thereafter during estrogen therapy.

Follow-up Tests

Annual tests which should be performed include:

- Pap smear in patients with uterus
- Bimanual examination
- Rectal examination

Semiannual tests which should be performed include:

- Blood pressure
- Hemoglobin
- Breast examination

Mammography

Any abnormality of the breasts requires prompt evaluation by mammography and/or direct biopsy. Likewise, any changes in mammary tissue require immediate evaluation. Breast self-examination should be taught to patients and recommended monthly. Semiannual breast exams should be done by the physician, more often if palpable abnormalities are present.

The American Cancer Society's guidelines on mammography should be followed. For normally palpable breasts, a baseline mammogram should be obtained:

- Between ages 35 and 40
- Every 2 years after the age of 40
- Annually after the age of 50

Estrogen therapy does not increase the risk for breast cancer (see Section #19), but postmenopausal women are reaching the age where the incidence of breast cancer continuously increases.

Diagnosis

The diagnosis of menopause can usually be made by history and physical examination, including vaginal hormonal cytology and the progestogen challenge test. If still uncertain, the best single laboratory test is serum FSH.

Postmenopausally, serum FSH and LH values are markedly elevated with FSH in the range of 75 to 200 mIU/ml, and LH in the range of 60 to 90 mIU/ml. Within a year after menses cease, serum FSH may increase as much as 13-fold, while LH rises approximately 3-fold. After a further rise in both FSH and LH during the early postmenopausal years, there is a gradual decline with age.

Thirty years after menopausal onset, serum gonadotrophin levels are only 40% to 50% of the maximum reached; however, these levels are still much higher than those found during the reproductive years. Serum FSH is more reliable for diagnosis of menopause since it usually rises more quickly and to higher levels than LH. Also, the mid-cycle LH surge in ovulating women could be mistaken for a postmenopausal level.

Serum estrogen levels are unreliable for diagnosis of menopause since the range of normal is so wide. Serum estradiol varies from 5-25 pg/ml after menopause and from 25-75 pg/ml in the follicular phase of reproductive-age women. Even total urinary estrogens cannot be used since post-menopausal values are 5 to 15 micrograms per 24 hours, compared to 10 to 25 micrograms per 24 hours during the follicular phase in ovulatory women. Estrogen levels in perimenopausal women should not be used for diagnosis; peaks and valleys occur in estrogen levels as ovarian function decreases.

#12 Oral Estrogens

Clinical Information

When the uterus is present, patients with menopausal symptoms should be prescribed estrogens and progestogens after proper evaluation (see Section #11) and in the absence of contraindications (see Section #25).

Dosages

Cyclic therapy is usually recommended to minimize side effects. However, continuous estrogen therapy is just as safe as long as the estrogen is opposed by a progestogen. Conjugated estrogens 0.625 mg, or equivalent dosages of other natural estrogens (see Table 1), can be given according to the calendar from the 1st through the 25th of the month. The progestogen should be added during the last 13 days of estrogen therapy, from the 13th through the 25th (see Table 5). If symptoms recur on the days off estrogens, continuous therapy can be used as long as the estrogen is opposed by a progestogen.

Although lower dosages are available, 0.625 mg of conjugated estrogens is the dosage that has been shown to prevent osteoporosis in 90% of postmenopausal women. Since prevention of osteoporosis is the major goal of estrogen replacement therapy, this is the lowest dosage that should be used.

After 2 to 3 months of estrogen therapy, if symptoms such as hot flushes persist, the estrogen dosage can be increased from 0.625 mg to 0.9 mg or to 1.25 mg of conjugated estrogens. It is rarely necessary to go above 1.25 mg to relieve menopausal symptoms. It is advisable to add an

12.

54

androgen (see Section #14) rather than continually increasing the estrogen dose.

Exceptions

There are two exceptions to the normal 0.625 mg dosage. These are women who:

- Have had surgical menopause during the reproductive years
- Have osteoporosis

Women with surgical menopause whose ovaries are removed during the reproductive years usually require higher dosages of conjugated estrogens, such as 1.25 mg, to relieve menopausal symptoms. However, after 1 to 2 years, this can usually be reduced to 0.625 mg.

Women with osteoporosis also need higher dosages, from 1.25 to 2.5 mg of conjugated estrogens, to reduce fracture rates.

Summary

It is sometimes more difficult to evaluate the patient who has had a hysterectomy and to initiate proper estrogen therapy. If bilateral oophorectomy was also performed during the reproductive years, estrogen therapy should be initiated soon after oophorectomy and the higher dosage of 1.25 mg conjugated estrogens is often required for prevention of symptoms.

When the ovaries are preserved, menopausal symptoms are commonly delayed until the expected time of natural menopause. However, after a hysterectomy, the ovaries may not continue to function fully until the expected age of natural menopause. Patients presenting with obvious vasomotor symptoms and/or atrophic vaginitis should be started on cyclic estrogen therapy with 0.625 mg of conjugated estrogens from the 1st through the 25th of the month.

For women who have had a hysterectomy and conservation of the ovaries with minimal symptoms, vaginal hormonal cytology and serum FSH may aid in diagnosis. To prevent osteoporosis, estrogen therapy can be instituted when hormonal evidence of menopause exists. In addition, from the 13th through the 25th of the month, cyclic progestogens should be added to the estrogen therapy for additional protection of the bones (see Section #5) and the breasts (see Section #19).

TABLE 1
ORAL ESTROGENS

NAME	ESTROGEN	MG	MANUFACTURER
Premarin	Conjugated Estrogens	0.3 0.625 0.9 1.25 2.5	Ayerst
Estrace	Micronized Estradiol	1.0 2.0	Mead Johnson
Estratab	Esterified Estrogens	0.3 0.625 1.25 2.5	Reid-Rowell
Ogen	Estropipate	0.625 1.25 2.5 5.0	Abbott
Estinyl	Ethinyl Estradiol	0.02 0.05 0.5	Schering
Estrovis	Quinestrol	0.1	Parke-Davis

#13 Non-Oral Estrogens

Estrogen Vaginal Cream

Vaginal cream is the longest available and is probably the most useful of the non-oral estrogens. Estrogens are well-absorbed through the vaginal mucosa so that good systemic levels are obtained in addition to local effects. Vaginal cream probably provides the quickest response and subsequent relief of symptoms of atrophic vaginitis, such as:

- Vaginal irritation
- Pruritus
- Vaginal dryness
- Dyspareunia

One common course of treatment is to apply Premarin vaginal cream, one gram daily (see Table 2). Usually, oral estrogens are started simultaneously. After 2 weeks of this double therapy, the maintenance dosage of the vaginal cream can often be reduced to 3 times weekly or entirely eliminated.

However, some patients on oral estrogens may continue to require estrogen vaginal cream for maintenance of the vaginal mucosa. Also, some women may not respond adequately to oral estrogens alone, developing dryness or pruritus of the vagina while on therapy. Instead of increasing the oral estrogen dosage, these women frequently benefit more from the addition of estrogen vaginal cream to the therapeutic routine.

Use of oral estrogens has been questioned because of portal absorption and liver metabolism as well as the risk of cholelithiasis. With the first liver pass, hepatic enzymatic changes may be induced that alter various biochemical parameters (Ref 13).Oral therapy may result in estrogen being delivered directly into hepatic tissue via the portal circulation. This could possibly result in changes in the rates of synthesis of certain hepatically-derived proteins and globulins such as:

- Renin substrate
- Cortisol binding globulin (CBG)
- Sex hormone binding globulin (SHBG)
- Ceruloplasmin
- Anti-thrombin III

Most of these changes are minor and may not be clinically significant.

Non-oral routes of administration deliver the estrogen directly into the systemic circulation and thus may cause less marked changes in hepatic biosynthesis because the portal system is by-passed. However, at least one of the benefits of oral therapy, the increase in HDL cholesterol, may be lost by non-oral administration. Apparently, the first liver pass is necessary to induce this anti-atherogenic lipoprotein.

Saturated Vaginal Rings

Silastic vaginal rings can be saturated with sex steroids, releasing fairly constant amounts of either estrogen and/or progestogen into peripheral blood. Whether this method will be widely accepted by patients remains to be determined, but cyclic therapy with the natural steroids — estradiol and progesterone — can be provided through the vaginal mucosa.

In contrast to oral micronized estradiol, vaginal estradiol:

- Provides a low estrone-to-estradiol ratio
- Does not induce a high postmedication estrogen peak
- Reaches the peripheral circulation without passing the enterohepatic circulation

Estradiol Subcutaneous Pellets

Subcutaneous implantation of 17beta-estradiol pellets, the principal human estrogen, has been available for over 50 years until temporarily banned by the FDA in 1980 for lack of efficacy and safety studies.

The main use of estradiol pellets has been in patients who could not use oral estrogens because of lack of response or side effects with oral estrogens. Estradiol pellets have been shown (Ref 79) to be very effective in relieving menopausal symptoms including:

- Hot flushes (or flashes)
- Insomnia
- Dyspareunia

Side effects, which occur in 5 to 8% of oral estrogen users, are diminished in those who use pellets because of simulation of the normal ovarian cycle.

When combined with subcutaneous testosterone pellets, estradiol implants are particularly effective in treating psychosexual problems such as loss of libido and anorgasmia, which may not respond to estrogen alone (Ref 39, 78). Estradiol pellets provide more normal estrone-to-estradiol ratios than oral estrogens and also provide more constant estrogen levels than any parenteral form of estrogen administration.

Transdermal Estradiol

The transdermal system of estrogen replacement therapy has recently been released for general clinical use. This system has been shown to be clinically effective in relieving menopausal symptoms. Comparative studies indicate that the transdermal system provides more normal estrone-to-estradiol ratios than oral estrogens.

Estraderm 0.05 mg or 0.1 mg daily elicited many of the desirable actions of estrogen while avoiding the pharmacologic effects of oral estrogens on hepatic proteins (Ref 12, 13). The patches are placed on the skin at 8 a.m. Monday and 8 p.m. Thursday, since estradiol levels are effective for 3½ days. The patch should be used continuously since symptoms may return when removed because of rapidly falling estradiol levels.

Although there are few or no undesirable effects, endometrial proliferation is normal and an oral progestogen must be given for 10 to 13 days. Transdermal estradiol does not produce as much of a rise in HDL cholesterol as oral estrogens and thus may not be as protective from atherosclerotic heart disease.

TABLE 2
ESTROGEN VAGINAL CREAM

NAME	ESTROGEN	MG/GM	MANUFACTURER
Premarin Vaginal Cream	conjugated estrogens	0.625 mg	Ayerst
Estrace Vaginal Cream	17beta-estradiol	0.1 mg	Mead Johnson
Ogen Vaginal Cream	estropipate	1.5 mg	Abbott
Ortho Dienestrol Cream	Dienestrol	0.01%	Ortho
Estragard Cream	Dienestrol	0.01%	Reid-Rowell
Diethylstilbestrol Suppositories	diethylstilbestrol	0.1 mg 0.5 mg	Lilly

TABLE 3

PARENTERAL ESTROGENS

NAME	ESTROGEN	MG/ML	MANUFACTURER
Depo-Estradiol	estradiol cypionate	1 mg 5 mg	Upjohn
Delestrogen	estradiol valerate	10 mg 20 mg 40 mg	Squibb
Estraval	estradiol valerate	10 mg 20 mg	Reid-Rowell
Estrapel*	estradiol pellet	25 mg pellet	Bartor, Progynon
Estraderm	transdermal estradiol	0.05 mg/day 0.1 mg/day	Ciba-Geigy

*Requires IND by FDA

#14 Androgens

Clinical Information

Estrogens give relief of most menopausal symptoms; however, it sometimes becomes necessary to add androgens to estrogen replacement therapy. Up to 75% of estrogen production is lost after menopause, but up to 50% of androgen production can also be lost when ovaries cease to function or are surgically removed. If symptoms persist, it is best to add a low dose of androgen to the estrogen replacement regimen rather than continue increasing the estrogen dosage beyond 1.25 mg of conjugated estrogens (see Table 4).

Potential benefits of androgens include alleviation of:

- Hot flushes (or flashes)
- Lethargy
- Endogenous depression
- Kraurosis vulvae (with use of 1-2% testosterone cream)
- Nocturia and incontinence
- Fibrocystic disease of the breast
- Headaches (migrainoid)

Although estrogens will alleviate both hot flushes and genital atrophy, the addition of an androgen will help overcome fatigue. When estrogens are contraindicated, as in patients with breast cancer, androgens alone may be helpful to relieve vasomotor symptoms and improve the psyche; however, they are of little value in treatment of genital atrophy and probably do not prevent osteoporosis in the dosages that can be used.

14

Some postmenopausal women complain of hirsutism before any hormone replacement. This is probably due to a relative imbalance of endogenous estrogens and androgens where estrogen levels decrease more than testosterone levels. Typically manifested by an increase in upper lip hair or small moustache, it usually lessens after estrogen replacement.

Androgen therapy can aggravate:

- Preexisting hirsutism
- Acne
- Skin oiliness

If there are good results from the androgen but aggravation of hirsutism or acne, reducing the androgen dosage and/or increasing the estrogen dosage may help. Spironolactone 25 mg q.i.d. may also be added to the estrogen-androgen combination so that the benefits of the androgen can be continued.

Research

In one study, relief of hot flushes was experienced by 96% with estradiol pellets, 89% with estradiol pellets plus testosterone, 55% with testosterone alone and 16% with placebo (Ref 39). Estrogen alone gave less benefit than estrogen-androgen pellets which:

- Increased feelings of well-being
- Improved libido
- Relieved endogenous depression
- Lessened migrainoid headaches

In postmenopausal women, androgens added to estrogen replacement commonly improve problems with:

- Libido
- Sexual response
- Anorgasmia

An increase in libido occurred in over 65% treated with androgens, 12.3% receiving estrogens and in only 1.8% taking the placebo (Ref 39).

In a study in which 76 women received pellet implants of either 50 mg of estradiol, a combination of 50 mg of estradiol and 100 mg of testosterone or placebo every 6 months, only those on the combination estrogen-androgen experienced a decided increase in sexual response and frequency of coitus (Ref 79, 80). The addition of testosterone implants also increased the frequency and intensity of orgasmic responses.

Recommendations

Available forms of androgen and estrogen/androgen combinations are found in Table 4.

ORAL THERAPY: Estratest or Estratest H.S. is a better-balanced combination than Premarin with methyl testosterone. Therapy should be cyclic from the 1st through the 25th of the month to minimize side effects and a progestogen should be added from the 13th through the 25th of the month. Although androgens may suppress the endometrium slightly, most patients on estrogen-androgen combination will have withdrawal menses from the progestogen challenge test.

INJECTABLES: Depo-Testadiol 1 cc i.m. will usually relieve symptoms for 4 weeks.

SUBCUTANEOUS PELLETS: Estradiol pellets are not available in the U.S. at this time. Testosterone pellets are the only form of androgen therapy available using the natural hormone, which reduces potential side effects. One or two 75 mg pellets of testosterone may be implanted subcutaneously, lasting 4-6 months, with the estrogen replacement given orally or by transdermal patch (Estraderm). Oral progestogens should also be added from the 13th to the 25th of the month.

TABLE 4
ANDROGENS

	NAME	ANDROGEN	MG/ML	MANUFACTURER
Oral Androgens	Oreton	methyl testosterone	5 mg	Schering
	Metandren	methyl testosterone	5 mg	Ciba
	Halotestin	fluoxymesterone	5 mg	Upjohn
	Fluoxymesterone	fluoxymesterone	5 mg	Reid-Rowell
Injectables	Depo-testosterone	testosterone cypionate	50 mg/ml	Upjohn
	Delatestryl	testosterone enanthate	100 mg/ml	Squibb
	Testopel	testosterone pellets	75 mg	Bartor
	Oreton	testosterone pellets	75 mg	Progynon

Estrogen/Androgen Combinations			
Estratest tablets	esterified estrogens methyl testosterone	1.25 mg 2.5 mg	Reid-Rowell
Estratest H.S. tablets	esterified estrogens methyl testosterone	0.625 mg 1.25 mg	Reid-Rowell
Premarin with Methyltestosterone	conjugated estrogens methyl testosterone	1.25 mg 10 mg	Ayerst
Premarin with Methyltestosterone	conjugated estrogens methyl testosterone	0.625 mg 5 mg	Ayerst
Depo-Testadiol	estradiol cypionate testosterone cypionate	2 mg 50 mg	Upjohn
Estrapel*	estradiol pellet (given with testosterone pellets)	25 mg	Bartor Progynon

*Requires IND by FDA

#15 Progestogens

Clinical Information

There are two ways that progestogens are commonly used in estrogen replacement therapy:

- Annually, in the progestogen challenge test
- Cyclically, to oppose estrogen effects

Progestogen Challenge Test

The progestogen challenge test should be performed on all climacteric women with an intact uterus who are:

- Asymptomatic, having a regular annual examination
- Symptomatic, being evaluated for estrogen therapy
- Currently on estrogen therapy, at annual examination

In the testing procedure, the patient takes 13 days of progestogen (see Table 5). If withdrawal bleeding occurs, progestogens should be added to the estrogen therapy from the 13th to the 25th of each monthly cycle. If there is no response, the progestogen challenge test should be repeated annually for asymptomatic women not using hormones.

Cyclic Use of Progestogens

Progestogens are increasingly being added to estrogen replacement therapy for postmenopausal women. In the 1970s, studies revealed that unopposed estrogen replacement increases the risk of endometrial cancer. Therefore, reasons for adding progestogens to estrogen replacement include:

15

- Prevention of endometrial cancer
- Reduction in risk of breast cancer
- Promotion of new bone formation
- Prevention and treatment of osteoporosis

Some troublesome effects of unopposed estrogen, such as breast tenderness, may be alleviated by adding progestogens. Although added progestogen may aggravate mastodynia when initiating therapy, this usually abates with time. Edema, bloating and irritability are more frequent in women using unopposed estrogens but are sometimes aggravated by added progestogen.

Other uses of progestogens during the climacteric include:

- Prevention of vasomotor flushes
- Avoidance of annual endometrial biopsies
- Decreasing the frequency of D&Cs performed for abnormal postmenopausal bleeding

One major drawback is that the same contraindications are listed for progestogens as for estrogens. However, this labeling should not preclude the physician from using his best judgment in the interest of the patient. There is no good evidence that progestogens have an adverse reaction on coagulation factors or mammary tissue in humans. There are also concerns about the long-term effects of progestogens, particularly with possible adverse effects on HDL cholesterol. Some patients are reluctant to resume menstruation and sometimes experience premenstrual-like symptoms during progestogen therapy. However, after menopause, menstrual effects are lessened for patients taking progestogens, including:

- Reduced menstrual flow (3-4 days)
- Lessened dysmenorrhea
- Lessened PMS

Research has demonstrated a reduction in abnormal postmenopausal bleeding. In one study, abnormal bleeding occurred in 23.3% of non-hormone users, 14.2% of users of estrogen alone and in only 3.9% of estrogen-progestogen users (Ref 34).

Although any unscheduled bleeding should be promptly investigated, annual endometrial biopsies are not required for users of progestogens. One study showed that hyperplasia or neoplasia occurred in 8.1% of non-hormone users, 7.9% of estrogen users and 0.9% of estrogen-progestogen users.

Adding Progestogen to Estrogen Replacement

Patients receiving oral estrogens from the 1st through the 25th of each month should have the progestogen added (see Table 5) from the 13th through the 25th for the benefit of the bones and the breasts (see Sections #5 and #18). This includes women who have had a hysterectomy.

Women on continuous estrogen, injectables or estradiol pellet implants, may be given the progestogen the first 13 days of each month.

For initial therapy, C-21 progestogens (such as Provera 10 mg) should be chosen for women with a past history of breast problems such as fibrocystic disease or mastodynia. 19-nor steroid progestogens (such as Aygestin 5 mg) are best for those with a past history of heavy or prolonged menstrual periods.

Studies show that less than 10 mg of Provera may not be protective for the endometrium (Ref 37, 90). Although 5 mg of Aygestin is the recommended starting dosage, as little as 1 mg of norethindrone may be protective for the endometrium. Injectable progestogens are not recommended for postmenopausal women with an intact uterus since the duration of action is irregular and breakthrough bleeding may result.

For continuous, low-dosage estrogen-progestogen therapy, it is recommended that Premarin (0.625 mg - 1.25 mg) and Provera (2.5 mg) be taken every day of the year. If breakthrough bleeding occurs, Provera should be increased to 5 mg. If after two weeks breakthrough bleeding continues, then Provera should be increased to 7.5 mg. With 0.625 mg Premarin, amenorrhea is immediate in 65% of patients. With 1.25 mg Premarin, amenorrhea is achieved by 47%.

Patients should be warned to expect irregular spotting the first 3-6 months of therapy.

Side Effects of Estrogen-Progestogen Therapy

The major side effect of estrogen-progestogen therapy is that 97% of patients have withdrawal bleeding until age 60, with 60% of patients continuing withdrawal bleeding after age 65. In addition, 5 to 10% of patients experience:

- Breast tenderness
- Edema
- Bloating
- Premenstrual irritability
- Lower abdominal cramps
- Dysmenorrhea

Patient acceptance of withdrawal bleeding has been good once the benefits are clearly explained. However, patients do not have to accept continued menses with alternative methods of combination estrogen-progestogen therapy (Ref 44).

Side effects may be managed by:

- Decreasing the estrogen dosage
- Adding a mild diuretic (HCTZ, 25 to 50 mg)
- Changing to another progestogen

For patients who cannot tolerate any oral progestogen, progesterone suppositories (25-50 mg daily) may be used.

General aches and pains can be dealt with by using a prostaglandin-inhibiting analgesic such as:

- Aspirin
- Motrin 400 to 800 mg q.i.d. (Ibuprofen, Upjohn)
- Naproxyn 250 to 500 mg t.i.d. (Naproxen, Syntex)
- Anaprox 275 mg t.i.d. (Naproxen Sodium, Syntex)
- Ponstel 250 mg q.i.d. (Mefenamic Acid, Parke-Davis)

TABLE 5
PROGESTOGENS

NAME	PROGESTOGEN	MG	MANUFACTURER
Provera	medroxyprogesterone acetate	10	Upjohn
Curretab	medroxyprogesterone acetate	10	Reid-Rowell
Cyrin	medroxyprogesterone acetate	10	Ayerst
Amen	medroxyprogesterone acetate	10	Carnrick
Aygestin	norethindrone acetate	5	Ayerst
Norlutate	norethindrone acetate	5	Parke-Davis
Norlutin	norethindrone	5	Parke-Davis
Megace	megesterol acetate	20	Bristol-Myers
		40	
Ovrette	norgestrel	0.075	Wyeth
Micronor	norethindrone	0.35	Ortho
Nor-Q.D.	norethindrone	0.35	Syntex
	Progesterone Vaginal Suppositories	25	—
		50	

#16 Calcium Supplements

Clinical Information

Bone loss due to osteoporosis is associated with alterations in calcium metabolism yielding negative calcium balance. Although calcium intake does not decrease at the time of menopause and calcium absorption does not vary greatly, a rise in fasting urinary calcium is found at about this time (Ref 23, 24).

As determined by the NIH Consensus Conference on Osteoporosis, the American diet is deficient in calcium intake, particularly among women who diet to maintain a thin figure (Ref 65). The usual daily intake of elemental calcium in the U.S., 450 mg to 550 mg, is below the National Research Council's recommended dietary allowance (RDA) of 800 mg. Calcium metabolic balance studies indicate a daily requirement of 1,000 mg of elemental calcium for premenopausal and estrogen-treated postmenopausal women. Postmenopausal women who are not treated with estrogens require 1,500 mg or more daily for calcium balance.

Calcium Level Changes

Changes in urinary calcium levels are difficult to detect since 24-hour collections reflect absorbed dietary calcium. Patients must be studied in a fasting state, when urinary calcium derives primarily from bone.

By comparing fasting calcium levels in hysectomized women who also had bilateral

oophorectomy to those who had ovarian conservation, the increase in resorption of calcium
from bone can be related to reduced ovarian estrogens (Ref 23). Both fasting plasma and urinary
hydroxyproline confirm that the increased calcium
excretion is due to increased bone resorption of
calcium. Women undergoing a natural menopause have similar changes in calcium metabolism. Postmenopausal women show a higher
morning fasting urinary calcium/creatinine ratio
than premenopausal women.

16

The increase in fasting serum or urinary calcium that follows either natural menopause or bilateral oophorectomy is reversible with estrogen
therapy. Estrogen administration also stimulates
calcitonin production, which is decreased after
menopause, and may affect bone calcium in-
directly since calcitonin is known to inhibit bone
resorption. Adding progestogens to estrogen
replacement therapy enhances the effects of the
estrogen, thereby promoting new bone formation
(Ref 84).

Recommendations

As recommended by the NIH Consensus
Conference on Osteoporosis, calcium supple-
ments are essential but of secondary importance
to estrogen replacement. Weight-bearing exercise was the third recommendation. A few studies have shown a reduction in fracture rate with
calcium alone; however, most studies have also
used estrogen replacement plus calcium.

Calcium carbonate is the most widely-studied
calcium and probably the best absorbed, with 40%
absorbed as elemental calcium. Other calcium

products can be used but amounts absorbed as elemental calcium vary. For example, only 10% of calcium lactate is absorbed as calcium. Most of the calcium makers now list the amount of elemental calcium in their products, not the total mg of calcium in each tablet (see Table 6).

Calcium supplementation should be started by age 35 to 40 since this is when women have peak bone mass. Women whose diets are markedly deficient in calcium should start supplementation earlier (Ref 65). The more bone mass a woman has entering menopause, the more she is apt to retain.

The major sources of calcium in the U.S. diet are milk and dairy products. Each 8 oz glass of milk contains 275 to 300 mg of calcium. Skim milk may actually contain more calcium. Other dietary sources of calcium include:

- Lowfat yogurt
- Cheese
- Fish, particularly those canned with bones
- Clams and oysters
- Spinach, broccoli, leafy vegetables
- Roasted peanuts with skins
- Tofu

Other agents that may be helpful in preventing osteoporosis include (Ref 3):

- Vitamin D or analogues
- Sodium fluoride
- Calcitriol
- Calcitonin
- Anabolic steroids
- Thiazide diuretics
- Magnesium

More research needs to be done with these agents before they can be widely recommended. Calcitonin (Calcimar, USV Laboratories) 100 IU daily subcutaneously or i.m. by injection is probably the best substitute for estrogen replacement when estrogens are contraindicated.

TABLE 6
CALCIUM SUPPLEMENTS

NAME	CALCIUM	ELEMENTAL CA	MANUFACTURER
Os-Cal 500	calcium carbonate	500 mg	Marion
Os-Cal 250	calcium carbonate + Vit D	250 mg	Marion
Posture	calcium phosphate	600 mg	Ayerst
Posture with D	calcium phosphate + Vit D	600 mg	Ayerst
Caltrate 600	calcium carbonate	600 mg	Lederle
Caltrate 600 + Vit D	calcium carbonate + Vit D	600 mg	Lederle
Citracal	calcium citrate	200 mg	Mission
Calcet	calcium lactate calcium gluconate calcium carbonate	152.8 mg	Mission
Tums	calcium carbonate	200 mg	Norcliff-Thager

Notes

#17 Endometrial Hyperplasia

Research

Hyperplasia of the endometrium has been established as a precancerous lesion in some women. In a prospective study of 562 women with adenomatous hyperplasia, 18.5% developed cancer after a few years, but by the 10th year the incidence of adenocarcinoma rose to 30% (Ref 41).

In another study, 115 patients with hyperplasia or adenocarcinoma-in-situ — were followed for two to eight years without any therapy, either hysterectomy or hormonal manipulation. A significant number developed invasive adenocarcinoma, including 26.7% of those with adenomatous hyperplasia, 81.8% of those with atypical hyperplasia and 100% of those with adenocarcinoma-in-situ (Ref 89).

Of the 31 patients with endometrial cancer in the Wilford Hall USAF Medical Center study, 11 (39.3%) had a previous diagnosis of hyperplasia from 4 months to 8 years before detection of cancer (Ref 32). Although earlier studies contend that adenomatous hyperplasia may be precancerous, any degree of hyperplasia may be significant since 6 of these 11 patients had only benign or cystic hyperplasia, yet developed endometrial cancer in a relatively short period of time.

In a 5-year prospective study, 325 women were found to have varying degrees of endometrial hyperplasia (Ref 32). They were treated with progestogens for 7 to 10 days each month for 3 to 6 months and curettage was repeated after therapy. Hyperplasia reversed to normal endometrium in 307 (94.5%). Of the 18 patients with persistent hyperplasia, 14 had been given progestogens for only 7 days each month and only 4 patients with persistent hyperplasia had been treated for 10 days monthly (see Table 7). For the past 5 years at the Medical College of Georgia, every endometrial hyperplasia has been successfully reversed to a normal endometrium within 6 months by using progestogens 13 days monthly.

Hyperplasia and ERT

Unopposed estrogens have a role in the development of endometrial hyperplasia and neoplasia, primarily because of incomplete shedding of the endometrium. Progesterone or progestogen therapy ensures more complete sloughing of the endometrium, leaving behind fewer glands and cells for continued proliferation and growth. The protective action of progestogens on the endometrium is primarily physical. However, additional actions of both natural progesterone and synthetic progestogens may be important (Ref 90). Progestogens decrease estrogen receptors in endometrial cells and induce estradiol dehydrogenase and isocitrate activity, which is the mechanism by whose means these cells metabolize estrogens.

Recommendations for Treatment

The preferred method of treatment for endometrial hyperplasia is an initial curettage followed by a course of progestogen therapy (see Table 4). Norlutate 5 mg or Provera 10 mg should be taken for 13 days monthly. After 6 months of progestogen therapy, the curettage should be repeated. If the endometrial hyperplasia is persistent, hysterectomy is recommended.

If the patient is on estrogen therapy, discontinuance is not necessary during the 6 months of progestogen therapy. The hyperplasia will reverse equally well on combined estrogen-progestogen therapy.

TABLE 7
EFFECTS OF PROGESTOGENS ON ENDOMETRIAL HYPERPLASIA
TOTAL NUMBER OF PATIENTS: 325

PATHOLOGY BEFORE THERAPY	NO. OF PATIENTS
Benign hyperplasia	196
Cystic hyperplasia	34
Adenomatous hyperplasia	28
Atypical adenomatous hyperplasia	67

ENDOMETRIUM AFTER THERAPY	
Proliferative	156
Secretory	69
Atrophic	53
Dyssynchronous maturation	29
Benign hyperplasia	12
Adenomatous hyperplasia	4
Atypical adenomatous hyperplasia	2

#18 Endometrial Cancer

Clinical Information

Unopposed estrogen therapy increases the risk of endometrial cancer, although the magnitude has been exaggerated by the methodology used in retrospective studies (Ref 56, 73, 75, 94). Progestogen added 10 to 13 days per month to estrogen replacement therapy reduces the risk of endometrial adenocarcinoma to less than that of untreated women (Ref 28, 31, 36, 43, 81, 82, 90). For those not needing estrogen replacement, use of the progestogen challenge test to screen

Incidence of Endometrial Cancer

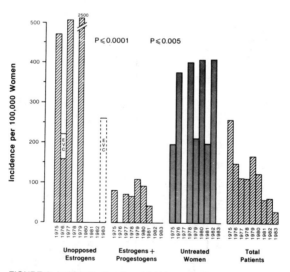

FIGURE 3. Incidence of endometrial cancer in the various treatment groups compared with untreated from 1975-1983 (Reproduced with permission from Gambrell) (Ref 32).

asymptomatic postmenopausal women can reduce adenocarcinoma of the endometrium (Ref 28).

Not all postmenopausal women need estrogens. Many produce sufficient endogenous estrogens to remain asymptomatic and prevent the metabolic changes of long-term estrogen deficiency in later life. However, within this group may be those in need of progestogens to prevent endometrial hyperplasia, possibly leading to endometrial carcinoma. The progestogen challenge test (see Section #15) was devised to identify those in this high risk group. A positive response to this test (withdrawal bleeding) indicates that 13 days per month of progestogen therapy should be continued for as long as withdrawal bleeding occurs in order to ensure complete endometrial shedding.

18.

Research

During the 5 years of prospective study and 4 years of follow-up at Wilford Hall USAF Medical Center from 1975-1983 (Figure 3), 5,563 postmenopausal women were registered in the hormone user survey (Ref 32). However, approximately 40% had a hysterectomy and consequently were not at risk for endometrial cancer. Adenocarcinoma of the endometrium was diagnosed in 31 patients during 27,243 patient-years of observation, for an overall incidence of 113.8 per 100,000 women per year (see Table 8).

The largest group of patients, the estrogen-progestogen users with 16,327 patient-years of observation, was found to have 8 cancers for an annual incidence of 49.0 per 100,000 women. The highest incidence of endometrial carcinoma was observed in the unopposed estrogen users, in whom 10 cancers were detected during 2,560 patient-years for an incidence of 390.6 per 100,000 women. The second highest incidence was 11 cancers in the nonhormone users during 4,480 patient-years of observation, for an incidence of 245.5 per 100,000 women. Only 2 endometrial cancers were observed in the estrogen vaginal cream users and no malignancies occurred in either the progestogen or androgen users. This group consisted primarily of progestogen users, women who had been identified as being at increased risk for adenocarcinoma by the progestogen challenge test and who were being treated with cyclic progestogens only.

Other studies have demonstrated the efficacy of progestogens in protecting estrogen users from adenocarcinoma. One reported no endometrial cancers in 72 estrogen-progestogen users but 11 cancers in 207 patients treated with unopposed estrogens (Ref 43). In a double-blind study, no adenocarcinomas were diagnosed in the 84 patients using estrogen-progestogen for 10 years, but 1 endometrial cancer occurred in the 84 placebo users (Ref 60). Studies from England have not uncovered any increased risk for endometrial malignancy in estrogen-treated postmenopausal women because they routinely add a progestogen (Ref 81, 83, 90). However, a 15% endometrial hyperplasia rate was observed in the unopposed estrogen users before progestogens were added (Ref 83).

TABLE 8

INCIDENCE OF ENDOMETRIAL CANCER AT WILFORD HALL USAF MEDICAL CENTER: 1975-1983

THERAPY GROUP	PATIENT-YEARS OF OBSERVATION	PATIENTS WITH CANCER	INCIDENCE (PER 100,000)
Estrogen-Progestogen Users	16,327	8	49.0
Unopposed Estrogen Users	2,560	10	390.6
Estrogen Vaginal Cream Users	2,716	2	73.6
Progestogen Users	1,160	0	—
Non-Users	4,480	11	245.5
TOTAL	27,243	31	113.8

#19 Breast Cancer

Clinical Information

Breast cancer is the most frequent malignancy in females, representing 28% of all cancers (Figure 4). In 1988, it was estimated that 142,000 new cases of breast cancer would be diagnosed during 1989 (Ref 1). The incidence of breast cancer increases throughout the female life span and it is estimated that one out of every ten women in the U.S. will eventually develop breast cancer.

There is no increased risk of breast cancer in estrogen users.

Research

Studies of both endometrial and breast cancer in estrogen users have indicated a modest association between unopposed estrogen therapy and adenocarcinoma of the endometrium. However, in every instance the association between estrogens and carcinoma of the breast was considerably less (Ref 28).

Only three studies have observed any significantly increased risk of breast cancer from estrogen therapy, and in all the only increased risk occurred in small subgroups of hormone users (Ref 47, 48, 69). In one of these studies, although the risk of breast cancer was significantly increased (RR = 1.59, 95% CI 1.18-2.10), the mortality from breast cancer in the estrogen users was significantly decreased (RR = 0.55, 95% CI 0.28-0.96) (Ref 47). In another study, four cases of breast cancer were found among 301 estrogen users followed for 5 to 25 years; an equal number

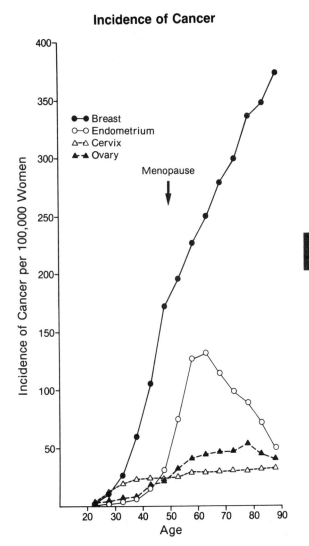

FIGURE 4. Incidence of breast, endometrial, cervical, and ovarian cancer in women by age (Reproduced with permission from Gambrell) (Ref 26).

was observed in the 309 nonusers (Ref 43). In a double-blind study, four breast cancers were detected in the 84 placebo users and none in the 84 estrogen-progestogen users ($P \leq 0.05$) (Ref 60).

A recent case-control study failed to show any significant risk for carcinoma of the breast from estrogen therapy for any duration or for any dose, whether or not the patient had ovaries (Ref 50). A significantly decreased risk of breast cancer was observed in 2 subgroups of estrogen users: in those with a family history of breast cancer, the relative risk (RR) was decreased to 0.2; and in those whose first term pregnancy was before age 20, the RR was reduced to 0.1. In a study from the CDC, the risk of breast cancer did not appear to increase with increasing duration of estrogen or latency, even for durations and latencies of twenty years or longer (Ref 92). This has also been confirmed by a recent study from Australia (Ref 68). Therefore, numerous long-term studies of large numbers of women have failed to incriminate estrogen replacement for any significantly increased risk of breast cancer.

During the 9 years of study and follow-up at Wilford Hall from 1975-1983, 69 postmenopausal women were diagnosed with breast cancer (Ref 32). With 48,669 patient-years of observation, the overall incidence of breast cancer was 141.8 per 100,000 women per year (see Table 9). The lowest incidence of mammary malignancy was observed in estrogen-progestogen users, with 11 cancers during 16,466 patient-years of observation for an annual incidence of 66.8 per 100,000 women. During 19,676 patient-years of unopposed estrogen use, there were 28 cancers for an incidence of 142.3 per 100,000. The incidence in nonusers with 22 carcinomas of the breast during 6,404 patient-years of observation, was 343.5 per 100,000.

There are at least two other studies which indicate that adding progestogen to estrogen replacement may actually decrease the risk for carcinoma of the breast. In the double-blind study, there were no breast cancers in the 84 estrogen-progestogen users while 4 were detected in the 84 placebo users, statistically significant with $P \leq 0.05$ (Ref 60). Another study observed a lower incidence of breast cancer in unopposed estrogen users (123 per 100,000) when compared to non-users (154 per 100,000), although this was not statistically significant (Ref 52). The incidence of mammary malignancy in the estrogen-progestogen users (109 per 100,000) was significantly lower ($P \leq 0.05$) when compared to either the estrogen users or nonusers. In the Wilford Hall study (Figure 5), the difference in the estrogen-progestogen users (66.8 per 100,000) and the nonusers (343.5 per 100,000) was statistically significant with $P \leq 0.01$. This incidence was also significantly lower than expected when compared to both the Third National Cancer Survey (188.3 per 100,000) and NCI SEER data (229.2 per 100,000) with $P \leq 0.01$.

Progesterone deficiency may increase the risk for breast cancer. In a long-term follow-up of a group of infertility patients, those with pro-gesterone deficiency had 5.4 times the risk of pre-menopausal carcinoma of the breast when compared with women in the nonhormone group (Ref 17). The incidence of postmenopausal breast cancer did not differ significantly between the two groups; however, these patients were just reaching menopause. Another study of progesterone deficiency did observe an increased risk of post-menopausal breast cancer (Ref 16). Chronic anovulation increased the risk of endometrial cancer 5-fold, and the risk for breast carcinoma after the age of 55 was increased 3.6-fold.

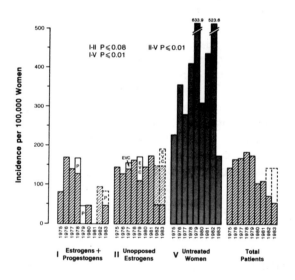

FIGURE 5. Incidence of breast cancer in the various treatment groups compared with untreated from 1975-1983 (Reproduced with permission from Gambrell) (Ref 32).

96

TABLE 9

INCIDENCE OF BREAST CANCER AT
WILFORD HALL USAF MEDICAL CENTER: 1975-1983

THERAPY GROUP	PATIENT-YEARS OF OBSERVATION	PATIENTS WITH CANCER	INCIDENCE (PER 100,000)
Estrogen-Progestogen Users	16,466	11	66.8
Unopposed Estrogen Users	19,676	28	142.3
Estrogen Vaginal Cream Users	4,298	5	116.3
Progestogen Users	1,825	3	164.4
Non-Users	6,404	22	343.5
TOTAL	48,669	69	141.8

#20 Thromboembolic Disease

Clinical Information

Estrogen replacement therapy has been thought to increase thromboembolic phenomena, which are listed as contraindications. This concept is largely based on observations suggesting an association between oral contraceptives and vascular thrombosis. Despite a positive association between aging and thrombolic complications, clinical studies have failed to observe any increased risk of these disorders (Ref 8, 42, 60, 62).

Coagulation changes which occur with aging include:

- Increase in factor V
- Increase in factor VII
- Possible increase in factor VIII
- No change in antithrombin III

Coagulation changes which occur with estrogen replacement include:

- Increase in fibrinogin (still within normal range)
- Slight decrease in antithrombin III (still within normal range)
- Decrease in factor V
- No change in factors VII or X
- No change in prothrombin time or partial thromboplastin time

Research

In one study, deaths from cerebral vascular accidents (CVA) declined from an expected 15 to

8 during estrogen therapy over a 15-year period of treatment (Ref 8). It was concluded that estrogens delay aging of the arteries. Although another recent study observed an increase in CVA, the only significant increase was in women who smoked (Ref 91). Another study found a significantly lower incidence of stroke syndromes in long-term estrogen users when compared with a similar group who had not used estrogens (Ref 42). No significant difference in the incidence of either thrombophlebitis or embolism was observed between estrogen-treated women and patients who had never received estrogens. In a double-blind study, thrombophlebitis occurred in 13 of 84 estrogen-progestogen users and 17 of 84 placebo users (Ref 60). Only one incidence of pulmonary embolism was encountered during the 10 years of this study and it occurred in a placebo user.

Estrogen labeling has been recently changed so that no longer are all thromboembolic events a contraindication. Active thrombophlebitis or thromboembolic disorders remain a contraindication as does a past history of thrombophlebitis, thrombosis or thromboembolic disorders associated with previous estrogen use. No longer are postpartum, postoperative or traumatic blood clots a contraindication. However, in patients with any history of thromboembolic disease, it would seem prudent to obtain coagulation studies before therapy and repeat these after three to six months of estrogen use.

#21 Hypertension

Research

Because the original high-dosage oral contraceptives caused transient hypertension in some young women, estrogen replacement therapy has been expected to have a similar effect. However, numerous studies have indicated that estrogen therapy has a beneficial effect on hypertension.

Some of these studies and their findings include:

- Duke University — incidence of new hypertensive cardiovascular disease 16.3% in estrogen-treated women vs. 31.7% in nonusers ($P \leq 0.001$) (Ref 42)
- Southern California — study of 1,496 women, after adjusting for effects of obesity, found estrogen-treated women tended to have lower blood pressure and blood glucose than controls (Ref 5)
- Wilford Hall — estrogen users had lower diastolic BP than other groups; nonusers were more obese ($P \leq 0.05$) (Ref 35)
- Australian studies observed a lowered systolic BP with one natural estrogen (Ogen) and lowered diastolic BP with another (Premarin) (Ref 93)
- An English study observed that both systolic and diastolic BP are significantly reduced in women on various regimens of hormone replacement (Ref 53)

Hypertension increases in the age group of postmenopausal women; cases will therefore be found among estrogen users (Ref 61, 86). However, these do not establish the role of estrogens in hypertension. Elevations in BP can coexist with hormone replacement, so blood pressure should be routinely monitored.

Other studies have reported on the effect of estrogen use on the renin-aldosterone system. One study showed no activation of the renin-aldosterone system in patients using estradiol valerate therapy (Ref 66). Another study reported an increased plasma renin activity in users of conjugated estrogens, but no effect on the renin concentration itself (Ref 64). Neither study observed any adverse effect of estrogens on blood pressure when hormone users were matched to controls and corrected for age and weight.

Recommendations for Treatment

If hypertension does occur in estrogen users, estrogen replacement does not have to stop (Ref 88). Instead, as a first step, salt intake should be restricted to 3,000 mg daily. If salt restriction alone does not control the hypertension, a mild antihypertensive such as hydrochlorothiazide (25-50 mg daily) can be added. Only if these two measures fail to improve blood pressure levels should there be consideration of ending estrogen replacement. Most antihypertensive patients require less medication after hormone replacement.

#22 Gallbladder Disease

Research

Some studies have indicated that estrogen replacement therapy increases the risk of gallbladder disease, especially cholelithiasis. The liver responds to oral estrogens by an increase in SHBG. It has been suggested that oral estrogens may affect the liver's excretory functions and may increase the incidence of gallstones.

Gallstones seem to occur more frequently in the silent form. In one study, oral cholecystography showed that 5.1% of those tested had gallstones present (Ref 70). Silent cases occurred twice as often and the diet was not significantly different in those with or without gallstones.

One evaluative study reported that the risk of surgically-confirmed gallbladder disease increased 2.5 times with estrogen therapy (Ref 6). In another study, the risk of cholesterol cholelithiasis was increased by both estrogens and obesity (Ref 46). Both factors operated independently with estrogen increasing the risk of gallstones at all weight levels. However, in the Duke University study, new occurrence of gallbladder disease was significantly lower ($P \leq 0.05$) in the estrogen users as compared with the controls (Ref 42). At the end of a 10-year New York study, the estrogen-progestogen group had a higher, although statistically insignificant, incidence of cholelithiasis (Ref 60).

The most recent study found no increased risk for gallstones among estrogen users (RR = 1.18, 95% CI 0.65-2.13) (Ref 49). Among estrogen users, the duration of use was similar in cases and controls.

Recommendations for Treatment

Since it is not feasible to screen all postmenopausal women for occult gallbladder disease prior to estrogen therapy, it has been suggested that patients should be instructed about the early signs of cholelithiasis (Ref 46). They are:

- Right upper quadrent pain
- Indigestion
- Eructation
- Nausea

22.

#23 Lipid Metabolism

Changes in Blood Lipid Profile

Both surgical and natural menopause appear to be related to adverse changes in blood lipid profile. These include:

- Development of atherosclerosis at an earlier age
- Increased hypertension
- Increased incidence of coronary artery disease

Natural Estrogens

Low dosages of natural estrogens increase HDL cholesterol with corresponding decreases in both LDL and very low density lipoproteins (VLDL), an antiatherogenic pattern (see Table 10) (Ref 13, 33).

The new transdermal estradiol system does not seem to be as effective in increasing HDL cholesterol as oral estrogens. Since the estradiol is absorbed directly into the blood, it avoids the first liver pass (Ref 12, 13).

In the Coronary Drug Project , high dosages of conjugated estrogens, 5-15 mg, had the opposite effect of lower dosages resulting in an atherogenic pattern of decreased HDL, with corresponding increases of both LDL and VLDL (Ref 15).

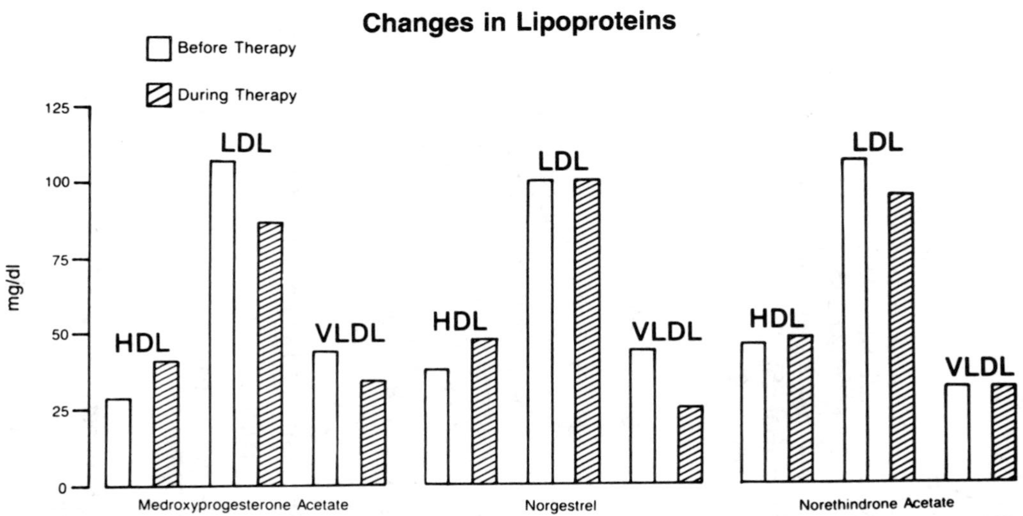

FIGURE 6. Changes in various fractions of lipoproteins with estrogen therapy combined with 3 different progestogens (HDL = high-density-lipoprotein; LDL = low-density lipoprotein; VLDL = very-low-density lipoprotein) (Reproduced with permission from Gambrell) (Ref 27).

Birth Control Pills

Moderate-to-high dosage oral contraceptives, such as 50 micrograms of ethinyl estradiol, increase both HDL and VLDL. However,
when the 19-nortestosterone progestogens are
added, the atherogenic pattern develops with a
decrease in HDL while LDL and VLDL both increase. HDL is further decreased by smoking and
results in a relative risk of 2.5 for heart disease
mortality (Ref 58). The newer low dosage birth
control pills do not have as much adverse effect on
lipid metabolism.

Added Progestogens

Although natural estrogens in low dosages
beneficially increase HDL cholesterol, added 19-
nortestosterone progestogens such as norgestrel
or norethinedrone acetate may negate this effect.
Ongoing studies at the Medical College of Georgia
compared effects of three different progestogens
added to estrogen replacement (Figure 6). These
were:

- Progesterone-like derivative Provera 10 mg

  ↑HDL   ↓LDL   ↓VLDL

- 19-nortestosterone derivative norgestrel
  0.075 mg

  ↑HDL   ~ LDL   ↓VLDL

- 19-nortestosterone derivative norethindrone
  acetate 5 mg

  ↑HDL   ↓LDL   ~VLDL
  (slight)   (moderate)

In all instances, the HDL-to-LDL ratio was improved, although Provera gave the most favorable lipid pattern. The added progestogen does not provide the increased HDL cholesterol, but it does not negate the estrogen-induced HDL. However, a comparative study between conjugated estrogens and injectable progestogen indicated that the favorable change in lipid pattern was similar (Ref 4). Either the estrogen or progestogen when used alone produced a significant decrease in total cholesterol, primarily by decreasing LDL. HDL cholesterol increased with both but the increase was not statistically significant with the progestogen. Since lower dosages of the 19-nortestosterone progestogens may be just as protective of the endometrium (Ref 90), lipid patterns may be equally favorable when dosages of these progestogens are reduced.

The tremendous benefit of preventing cardiovascular disease from postmenopausal estrogen use cannot be fully explained by the changes in lipid pattern (Ref 33). Other factors have a role such as a direct effect of estrogens upon arterial walls since estrogen receptors have been identified in coronary vessels. Favorable changes in prostocyclin and thromboxane metabolism may also occur with estrogen use.

TABLE 10

CHANGES IN LIPOPROTEINS WITH VARIOUS SEX STEROIDS

STEROID	HDL	LDL	VLDL
Conjugated estrogens 2.5 mg	↑	→	→
Estradiol pellets	↑	→	→
Micronized estradiol	↑	→	→
Estradiol valerate 2 mg	↑	→	→
Estradiol valerate 4 mg	↑	○	↓
Ethinyl estradiol 20 μg	↑	○	○
Ethinyl estradiol 50 μg	↑	○	↓
Ethinyl estradiol + progestogen	↓	↓	↓
Conjugated estrogens 5 mg	↓	↓	↓

Notes

#24 Management of Side Effects

Resumption of Menses

In postmenopausal women treated with combination estrogen-progestogen therapy, withdrawal bleeding occurs in as many as 97% until age 60, decreasing to 60% after age 65.

Generally, patient acceptance of resumption of menses has been good if the relative benefits and risks are carefully explained, including:

- The reduced incidence of endometrial cancer (see Section #18)
- No increased risk of breast cancer; in some, added progestogen reduces incidence of breast cancer (see Section #19)
- Promotion of new bone formation, helping restore bone that has been lost to osteoporosis (see Section #5)

In addition, the menses often change for the better. Frequently, the menses:

- Are lighter
- Are less painful
- Have less abnormal bleeding

Patients most reluctant to resume menses are those who experienced adverse menstrual effects. After menopause, withdrawal menses from hormone therapy are usually:

- Only 3-4 days in duration
- Free of dysmenorrhea
- Without PMS

In one study (Ref 34), abnormal bleeding requiring curettage occurred in:

- 23.3% of non-hormone users
- 14% of unopposed estrogen users
- Only 3.9% of estrogen-progestogen users

In addition, the estrogen-progestogen users need not have the annual endometrial biopsies that are recommended for all unopposed estrogen users with an intact uterus (see Section #9).

For those patients who cannot tolerate resumption of menses, continuous low dosage estrogen-progestogen therapy is an alternative that will produce amenorrhea in 60% of patients after 4-6 months (see Section #15).

Side Effects of Estrogens

Side effects of estrogens may include:

- Breast tenderness
- Edema or bloating
- PMS-like symptoms
- Nausea
- Headaches

Most patients have few, if any, side effects from estrogen replacement. If side effects occur, they are minimal and transient.

24.

Breast tenderness and sometimes slight breast enlargement may occur during the first 2-3 months after initiation of therapy. Mastodynia usually abates with time; reassurance is often all that a patient needs. If breast tenderness persists, the estrogen dosage can be reduced if more than

0.625 mg conjugated estrogens were prescribed. However, this should be the lowest dosage in order to prevent osteoporosis (see Section #5).

Adding a progestogen to estrogen therapy reduces breast tenderness in time, although it may initially aggravate breast tenderness. Reassurance to the patient is often all that is needed. Adding androgens to estrogen therapy or to estrogen-progestogen therapy may also ameliorate breast tenderness.

A mild diuretic, such as hydrochlorothiazide (25-50 mg), will relieve symptoms caused by estrogen-related fluid retention such as:

- Edema
- Bloating
- Abdominal pressure
- Breast tenderness
- PMS-like symptoms (headache, irritability)

The diuretic is usually given 7 to 10 days before menses during the days of added progestogen. A change to a different estrogen is sometimes necessary (see Table 1) or a change in the route of administration, such as the new transdermal estrogen, may help.

Nausea is rare in the low dosages of estrogen usually required for estrogen replacement. If nausea persists after two months of therapy, a change of estrogens or the route of administration may help.

Headaches are generally relieved by estrogen replacement. Most headaches are transient and respond to analgesics. Others may occur only with cyclic therapy, on the days at the end of the month when estrogens are not taken. Estrogens can be taken continuously as long as they are opposed with progestogens for 13 days each month. Rarely, migraine or migrainoid headaches may occur with estrogen replacement. Sometimes headaches respond to a mild diuretic, but it may be necessary to add an androgen to the estrogen therapy. The best response is offered by combination products such as:

- Estratest (orally)
- Depo-Testadiol (by injection)
- Estradiol-testosterone pellets

Side Effects of Progestogens

Side effects of progestogens include:

- PMS-like symptoms
- Lethargy
- Depression and irritability
- Abdominal bloating
- Breast tenderness

Mild PMS-like symptoms usually respond to a diuretic such as hydrochlorothiazide, 25-50 mg for 7 to 10 days before menses. If this is ineffective, a change should be made to another oral progestogen.

Breast tenderness may be initiated, aggravated or relieved when progestogens are added to estrogen replacement. Symptoms usually abate after 3 to 6 months. If mastodynia persists, a change should be made to another progestogen (see Table 5). For some women, C-21 progestogens such as medroxyprogesterone acetate, are better than 19-nortestosterone progestogens, such as norethindrone acetate. For others, the reverse is true.

In a rare case, a woman may experience side effects with all oral progestogens. Progesterone vaginal suppositories (25-50 mg) often eliminate these reactions.

Notes

#25 Contraindications

Contraindications for Estrogens

The following contraindications are listed in the product literature for most estrogens:

- Known or suspected cancer of the breast
- Known or suspected estrogen-dependent neoplasia
- Known or suspected pregnancy
- Undiagnosed abnormal genital bleeding
- Active thrombophlebitis or thromboembolic disorders
- A past history of problems associated with previous estrogen use:
  - Thrombophlebitis
  - Thrombosis
  - Thromboembolic disorders

There is no evidence that estrogen replacement increases the risk for breast cancer. However, estrogens are the growth hormone of mammary tissue and these contraindications must be observed until further data is accumulated (see Section #19). Theoretically, estrogen receptors in carcinoma of the breast would allow selection of some patients for estrogen replacement, yet only 50% of estrogen receptor positive tumors will respond to either endocrine ablative surgery or antiestrogen therapy. When progesterone receptors in mammary cancer are also positive, this predictive response increases to 70%. However, it has not yet been determined which patients could be safely treated.

Endometrial cancer may not have to remain a strict contraindication. Gynecologic Oncology at Wilford Hall USAF Medical Center provided estrogen replacement in women with Stage I well-differentiated adenocarcinoma of the endometrium since there was little likelihood of metastases. The 5-year survival was in excess of 96.7%. A recent study from Duke University indicated that prognosis was actually improved in endometrial cancer patients treated with estrogens (Ref 18).

Any abnormal postmenopausal bleeding should be thoroughly evaluated (see Section #9). Once malignancy is excluded and endometrial hyperplasia has been adequately treated with progestogens (see Section # 17), estrogen-progestogen replacement therapy can be safely administered.

Although there is no evidence that low dosages of natural estrogens have any adverse effect on coagulation factors or thromboembolic disease (see Section #20), estrogen replacement should be withheld in women who had blood clots previously while using estrogens. Thromboembolic events not related to a past history of hormone use no longer are contraindications for replacement therapy.

Contraindications for Progestogens

The following contraindications are listed in the product literature for most progestogens:

- A past or present history of:
  - Thrombophlebitis
  - Thromboembolic disorders
  - Cerebral apoplexy
- Liver dysfunction or disease

25.

- Known or suspected carcinoma of the breast
- Undiagnosed vaginal bleeding
- Missed abortion
- As a diagnostic test for pregnancy

Almost identical contraindications are listed for progestogens as for estrogens, even though there is no evidence that progestogens have any adverse effect on coagulation factors or thromboembolic disorders. However, this labeling should not preclude the physician from using his best judgment in the interest of the patient.

If liver function studies are normal, a patient with a history of liver dysfunction or disease can safely be given progestogens; however, liver function studies should be repeated after 3 to 6 months of progestogen therapy.

There is no evidence that progestogens increase the risk for breast cancer. There is, in fact, increasing evidence that adding progestogens to estrogen replacement may decrease the risk for carcinoma of the breast in some women (see Section #19) and that long-term progesterone deficiency can increase the risk for breast cancer (Ref 16, 17). For medical/legal reasons, however, breast cancer must remain a strict contraindication for progestogen therapy.

Undiagnosed genital bleeding becomes diagnosed in the course of proper evaluation of postmenopausal women (see Section #9). Endometrial hyperplasia should be treated with progestogens to prevent adenocarcinoma of the endometrium.

Notes

#26 Alternative Therapy

Clinical Information

Estrogens and progestogens are always the preferred treatment since they not only relieve menopausal symptoms but also prevent the metabolic consequences — osteoporosis and atherosclerosis — of long-term estrogen deficiency. If estrogens are contraindicated, progestogens cannot be used since the contraindications are identical (see Section #25). Alternative therapies are available to treat menopausal symptoms, including:

- Vasomotor symptoms
- Urogenital atrophy
- Psychogenic manifestations
- Osteoporosis

Vasomotor Symptoms

Androgens are effective in relieving such symptoms as:

- Hot flushes (or flashes)
- Night sweats
- Psychogenic manifestations

Any of the oral androgens such as methyltestosterone 5 mg (see Table 4) or injectables such as Depo-testosterone (50 mg every 4 weeks) can be used. However, androgens do not prevent atrophic vaginitis or coronary artery disease and they are probably ineffective in preventing osteoporosis in the dosages that can be given to postmenopausal women.

Bellergal (by Sandoz) is a tablet combining phenobarbital, ergotamine and belladonnine alkaloids. It is effective for:

- Reducing hot flushes
- Reducing night sweats
- Helping to calm restlessness
- Relieving insomnia

The dosage is one tablet morning and noon followed by two tablets at bedtime. Bellergal-S is the long-acting form given b.i.d.

Clonidine HCL (Catapres, by Boehringer Ingelheim) is an antihypertensive agent effective for hot flushes. The dosage is 0.1 mg t.i.d.

Urogenital Atrophy

No good alternative to estrogen is available for treatment of atrophic vaginitis. If oral estrogens are contraindicated, so are estrogen vaginal creams, which are well absorbed through the vaginal mucosa. Local antibiotics will treat infections and 1-2% testosterone cream is effective for kaurosis vulvae. Surgical lubricants can be prescribed for dyspareunia.

Psychogenic Manifestations

Alternative therapy available for treatment of psychogenic manifestations include:

- Tranquilizers
- Androgens
- Calcium channel blockers

26.

Tranquilizers can be used to treat depression and restlessness, but they are not a good substitute for estrogen replacement since they do not prevent effects of menopausal estrogen deprivation.

Androgens are most effective when they can be prescribed along with estrogens. Used alone, androgens still offer:

- Treatment of disturbances of the libido
- Promotion of a sense of well-being
- Partial relief of depression

A calcium channel blocker, such as Verapamil HCL (Calan by Searle), can be fairly effective in relieving headaches. It works best when combined with estrogen replacement but can be effective used alone. The dosage is titrated, starting with 80 mg daily, increasing every week to a maximum of q.i.d. until headaches are blocked.

Osteoporosis and Atherosclerosis

When estrogens are contraindicated, calcium supplementation should be increased to 1,500 to 2,000 mg daily (see Section #16). There is some evidence that calcium alone will help to prevent osteoporosis and reduce fracture rate (Ref 67), although this has recently been questioned. It is best to provide estrogen replacement whenever possible.

In addition to these higher doses of calcium, calcitonin is probably the best preventative for osteoporosis when estrogens are contraindicated.

However, calcitonin is:

- Expensive
- In short supply, until recently
- Given by injection at least 3 times weekly

There is really no alternative to estrogen replacement for prevention of atherosclerosis. Good nutrition is advisable to reduce dietary intake of cholesterol. Other measures include recommendation of an increase in physical activity such as jogging or brisk walks.

References

1. American Cancer Society: Cancer statistics, 1989. Ca-Cancer J Clinicians, 1989;39:3.

2. Anderson E, Hamburger S, Lin JH, et al: Characteristics of menopausal women seeking assistance. Am J Obstet Gynecol 1987;156:428.

3. Arnaud CD, Christiansen C, Cummings SR, et al: Consensus development conference: prophylaxis and treatment of osteoporosis. Br Med J 1987;295:914.

4. Barnes RB, Roy S, Lobo RA: Comparison of lipid and androgen levels after conjugated estrogen or depot-medroxyprogesterone acetate treatment in postmenopausal women. Obstet Gynecol 1985;66:216.

5. Barrett-Conner E, Brown V, Turner J, et al: Heart disease risk factors and hormone use in postmenopausal women. JAMA 1978;241:2167.

6. Boston Collaborative Drug Surveillance Program: Surgically confirmed gallbladder disease, venous thromboembolism and breast tumors in relation to postmenopausal estrogen therapy. N Engl J Med 1974;290:15.

7. Brown KH, Hammond CB: Urogenital atrophy. Obstet Gynecol Clinics N Am 1987;15:13.

8. Burch JC, Byrd BF, Vaughn WK: Results of estrogen treatment in one thousand hysterectomized women for 14,318 years. In Consensus on Menopausal Research, ed by van Keep PA, Greenblatt RB, Albeaux-Fernet M. Lancaster, England, MTP Press Ltd 1976;164.

9. Bush TL, Barrett-Connor E, Cowan LD, et al: Cardiovascular mortality and noncontraceptive use of estrogen in women: results from The Lipid Research Clinics Program follow-up study. Circulation 1987;75:1102.

10. Campbell S: Potency and hepato-cellular effects of oestrogens after oral, percutaneous, and subcutaneous administration. In The Controversial Climacteric, ed by van Keep PA, Utian WH, Vermeulen A. Lancaster, England, MTP Press Ltd 1982; 103.

11. Campbell S, Whitehead M: Oestrogen therapy and the menopausal syndrome. In Clinics in Obstetrics and Gynaecology, ed by Greenblatt RB, Studd JWW. London, England, WB Saunders Co, Ltd 1977;31.

12. Cedars MI, Judd HL: Nonoral routes of estrogen administration. Obstet Gynecol Clinics N Am 1987;14:269.

13. Chetkowski RJ, Meldrum DR, Steingold KA, et al: Biologic effects of transdermal estradiol. N Engl J Med 1986;314:1615.

14. Christiansen C, Christensen MS, Transbol I: Bone mass in postmenopausal women after withdrawal of oestrogen/progestogen replacement therapy. Lancet 1981;1:459.

15. The Coronary Drug Project Research Group: The coronary drug project: Initial findings leading to modifications of its research protocol. JAMA 1970;214:1303.

16. Coulam CB, Annegers JF: Chronic anovulation may increase postmenopausal breast cancer risk. JAMA 1983;249:445.

17. Cowan LD, Gordis L, Tonascia JA, et al: Breast cancer incidence in women with a history of progesterone deficiency. Am J Epidemiol 1981;114:209.

18. Creasman WT, Henderson D, Hinshaw W, et al: Estrogen replacement therapy in the patient treated for endometrial cancer. Obstet Gynecol 1986;67:326.

19. Crilley RG, Marshall DH, Nordin BEC: The effect of oestradiol valerate and cyclic oestradiol valerate/DL-norgestrel on calcium metabolism. Postgrad Med J 1978;54:47.

20. Crona N, Enk L, Mattson LA, et al: Progestogens and lipid metabolism. Maturitas 1986;8:141.

21. Dennerstein L, Laby B, Burrows GD, et al: Headache and sex hormone therapy. Headache 1978;18:146.

22. Ettinger B, Genant HK, Cann CE: Long-term replacement therapy prevents bone loss and fractures. Ann Int Med 1985;102:319.

23. Gallagher JC, Riggs RL, Deluca HF: Effect of estrogen on calcium absorption and serum vitamin D metabolites in postmenopausal osteoporosis. J Clin Endocrinol Metab 1980;51:1359.

24. Gallagher JC, Horsman A, Nordin BEC: Osteoporosis and the menopause. In The Menopausal Syndrome, ed by Greenblatt RB, Mahesh VB, McDonough PG. New York, Medcom Press, 1974;38.

25. Gambrell RD Jr: The menopause: Benefits and risks of estrogen-progestogen replacement therapy. Fertil Steril 1982;37:457.

26. Gambrell RD Jr: Breast disease in the postmenopausal years. Seminar Reprod Endocrinol 1983;1:27.

27. Gambrell RD Jr: The menopause: Benefits and risks of estrogen-progestogen replacement therapy. IM-Int Med Specialists 1985;6:135.

28. Gambrell RD Jr: Prevention of endometrial cancer with progestogens. Maturitas 1986;8:159.

29. Gambrell RD Jr: Sex steroids and cancer. Obstet Gynecol Clin N Am 1987;14:191.

30.   Gambrell RD Jr: Hormone replacement therapy and breast cancer. Maturitas 1987;9:123.

31.   Gambrell RD Jr: Use of progestogen therapy. Am J Obstet Gynecol 1987;156:1304.

32.   Gambrell RD Jr: Studies of endometrial and breast disease with hormone replacement therapy. In The Menopause, ed by Studd JWW and Whitehead MI. Oxford, England: Blackwell Scientific Publication, Ltd 1988; 247-261.

33.   Gambrell RD Jr: Editorial: Progestogens and lipids. Maturitas 1988;10:175.

34.   Gambrell RD Jr, Castaneda TA, Ricci CA: Management of postmenopausal bleeding to prevent endometrial cancer. Maturitas 1978;1:99.

35.   Gambrell RD Jr, Maier RC, Sanders BI: Decreased incidence of breast cancer in postmenopausal estrogen-progestogen users. Obstet Gynecol 1983;62:435.

36.   Gambrell RD Jr, Massey FM, Castaneda TA, et al: Use of the progestogen challenge test to reduce the risk of endometrial cancer. Obstet Gynecol 1980;55:732.

37.   Gibbons WE, Moyer DL, Lobo RA, et al: Biochemical and histologic effects of sequential estrogen/progestin therapy on the endometrium of postmenopausal women. Am J Obstet Gynecol 1986;154:456.

38. Gordan GS: Drug treatment of the osteoporoses. Ann Rev Pharmacol Toxicol 1978;18:253.

39. Greenblatt RB: The use of androgens in the menopause and other gynecic disorders. Obstet Gynecol Clinics N Am 1987;14:251.

40. Gruchow HW, Anderson AJ, Barborink JJ, et al: Postmenopausal use of estrogen and occlusion of coronary arteries. Am Heart J 1988;115:954.

41. Gusberg SB: The individual at high risk for endometrial carcinoma. Am J Obstet Gynecol 1976;126:535.

42. Hammond CB, Jelovsek FR, Lee KL, et al: Effects of long term estrogen replacement therapy. I - Metabolic. Am J Obstet Gynecol 1979;133:525.

43. Hammond CB, Jelovsek FR, Lee KI, et al: Effects of long term estrogen replacement therapy. II - Neoplasia. Am J Obstet Gynecol 1979;133:537.

44. Hanna JH, Brady WK, Hill JM, et al: Detection of postmenopausal women at risk for endometrial carcinoma by a progesterone challenge test. Am J Obstet Gynecol 1983;147:872.

45. Henderson BE, Paganini-Hill A, Ross RK: Estrogen replacement therapy and protection from acute myocardial infarction. Am J Obstet Gynecol 1988;159:312.

46. Honore LH: Increased incidence of symptomatic cholesterol cholelithiasis in perimenopausal women receiving estrogen replacement therapy. J Reprod Med 1980;25:187.

47. Hunt K, Vessey M, McPherson K: Long-term surveillance of mortality and cancer incidence in women receiving hormone replacement therapy. Br J Obstet Gynaecol 1987;94:620.

48. Jick H, Walker AM, Watkins RN, et al: Replacement estrogens and breast cancer. Am J Epidemiol 1980;112:586.

49. Kakar F, Weiss NS, Strite SA: Noncontraceptive estrogen use and the risk of gallstone disease in women. Am J Public Health 1988;78:564.

50. Kaufman DW, Miller DR, Rosenberg L, et al: Noncontraceptive estrogen use and the risk of breast cancer. JAMA 1984;252:63.

51. Kay C: Present perspectives and clinical implications. J Obstet Gynaecol 1984;4S:S98.

52. Lauritzen C, Meier F: Risks of endometrial and mammary cancer morbidity and mortality in long-term estrogen treatment. In The Climacteric - An Update, ed by van Herendael H & B, Riphagen FE, Goessens L, van der Pas H. Lancaster, England, MTP Press Ltd 1984;207.

53. Lind T, Cameron FC, Hunter FM, et al: A prospective controlled trial of six forms of hormone replacement therapy given to postmenopausal women. Br J Obstet Gynaecol 1979;86:1.

54. Lindsay R: Prevention of postmenopausal osteoporosis. Obstet Gynecol Clinics N Am 1987;14:63.

55. Lindsay R, Hamet DM, Clark DM: The minimum effective dose of estrogens for prevention of postmenopausal bone loss. Obstet Gynecol 1984;63:759.

56. Mack TM, Pike MC, Henderson BE, et al: Estrogens and endometrial cancer in a retirement community. N Engl J Med 1976;294:1262.

57. Magos AL, Brincat M, Studd JWW, et al: Amenorrhea and endometrial atrophy following continuous oral estrogens and progestogen therapy in postmenopausal women. Obstet Gynecol 1985;65:496.

58. Mann JI, Vessey MP, Thorogood M, et al: Myocardial infarction in young women with special reference to oral contraceptive practice. Brit Med J 1975;2:241.

59. Nachtigall LE, Nachtigall RH, Nachtigall RB, et al: Estrogen replacement I: A 10-year prospective study in the relationship to osteoporosis. Obstet Gynecol 1979;53:277.

60. Nachtigall LE, Nachtigall RH, Nachtigall RB, et al: Estrogen replacement II: A prospective study in the relationship to carcinoma and cardiovascular and metabolic problems. Obstet Gynecol 1979;54:74.

61. Notelovitz M: Effect of natural oestrogens on blood pressure and weight in postmenopausal women. S Afr Med J 1975;49:2251.

62. Notelovitz M: Exercise, nutrition, and the coagulation effects of estrogen replacement on cardiovascular health. Obstet Gynecol Clin N Am 1987;14:121.

63. Padwick MC, Pryse-Davies J, Whitehead MI: A simple method for determining the optimal dosage of progestin in postmenopausal women receiving estrogens. N Engl J Med 1986;315:930.

64. Pallas KG, Holzwarth GJ, Stern MP, et al: The effect of conjugated estrogens on the renin-angiotensin system. J Clin Endocrinol Metab 1977;44:1061.

65. Peck WA, Barrett-Conner E, Buckwalter JA, Gambrell RD Jr., et al: Consensus conference; Osteoporosis. JAMA 1984;252:799.

66. Punnonen R, Lammintausta R, Erkkda R, et al: Estradiol valerate therapy and the renin-aldosterone system in castrated women. Maturitas 1980;2:91.

67. Riggs BL, Seeman E, Hodgson SF, et al: Effect of the fluoride-calcium regimen on vertebral fracture occurrence in postmenopausal osteoporosis. N Engl J Med 1982;306:446.

68. Rohan TE, McMichael AJ: Non-contraceptive exogenous oestrogen therapy and breast cancer. Med J Aust 1988;148:217.

69. Ross RK, Paganini-Hill A, Gerkins VR, et al: A case control study of menopausal estrogen therapy and breast cancer. JAMA 1980;243:1635.

70. Sarles H, Gerolami A, Cros RC: Diet and cholesterol gallstones: a further study. Digestion 1978;17:128.

71. Sarrel PM: Sexuality in the middle years. Obstet Gynecol Clinics N Am 1987;15:49.

72. Semmens JP, Wagner G: Estrogen deprivation and vaginal function in postmenopausal women. JAMA 1982;248:445.

73. Shapiro S, Kelly JP, Rosenberg L, et al: Risk of localized and widespread endometrial cancer in relation to recent and discontinued use of conjugated estrogens. N Engl J Med 1985;313:969.

74. Sherwin BB, Gelfund MM: Differential symptom response to parenteral estrogen and/or androgen administration in the surgical menopause. Am J Obstet Gynecol 1985;151:153.

75. Smith DC, Prentice R, Thompson DJ, et al: Association of exogenous estrogen and endometrial carcinoma. N Engl J Med 1975;293:1164.

76. Speroff L, Glass RH, Kase NG: Clinical Gynecologic Endocrinology and Infertility. Baltimore MD, Williams and Wilkins Co, 1983;101 & 552.

77. Stampfer MJ, Willett WC, Colditz GA, et al: A prospective study of postmenopausal estrogen therapy and coronary heart disease. N Engl J Med 1985,313:1044.

78. Studd JWW: The climacteric syndrome. In Female and Male Climacteric, ed by Serr DM, van Keep PA, Greenblatt RB. Lancaster, England, MTP Press Ltd 1979; 23.

79. Studd J, Magos A: Hormone pellet implantation for the menopause and premenstrual syndrome. Obstet Gynecol Clinics N Am 1987;14:229.

80. Studd JWW, Collins WP: Oestradiol and testosterone implants in the treatment of psychosexual problems in the postmenopausal woman. Br J Gynaecol 1977;84:314.

81. Sturdee DW, Wade-Evans T, Paterson MEL, et al: Relationship between bleeding pattern, endometrial histology and oestrogen treatment in menopausal women. Br Med J 1978;1:1575.

82. Sullivan JM, Zwagg RV, Lemp GF, et al: Postmenopausal estrogen use and coronary atherosclerosis. Ann Int Med 1988;108:358.

83. Thom MH, White PJ, Williams RM, et al: Prevention and treatment of endometrial disease in climacteric women receiving oestrogen therapy. Lancet 1979;2:455.

84. Upton GV: The perimenopause: Physiologic correlates and clinical management. J Reprod Med 1982;27:1.

85. Utian WH: Definitive symptoms of postmenopause — incorporating use of vaginal parabasal cell index. In Estrogens in the Post-Menopause, Vol 3, Frontiers of Hormone Research, ed by van Keep PA, Lauritzen C. Basel, Switzerland, Karger, 1975; 74.

86. Utian WH: Effect of postmenopausal estrogen therapy on diastolic blood pressure and body weight. Maturitas 1978;1:3.

87. Vanhulle, G, Demol R: A double-blind study into the influence of estriol on a number of psychological tests in post-menopausal women. In Consensus on Menopause Research, ed by van Keep PA, Greenblatt RB, Albeaux-Fernet M. Lancaster, England, MTP Press Ltd 1976;94.

88. von Eiff AW: Blood pressure and estrogens. Front Horm Res 1975;3:177.

89. Wentz WB: Progestin therapy in endometrial hyperplasia. Gynecol Oncol 1974;2:362.

90. Whitehead MI, Fraser D: The effects of estrogens and progestogens on the endometrium. Obstet Gynecol Clin N Am 1987;14:299.

91. Wilson PWF, Garrison RJ, Castelli WP: Postmenopausal estrogen use, cigarette smoking, and cardiovascular morbidity in women over 50. N Engl J Med 1985;313:1038.

92. Wingo PA, Layde PM, Lee NC, et al: The risk of breast cancer in postmenopausal women who have used estrogen replacement therapy. JAMA 1987;257:209.

93. Wren BO, Routledge AD: The effect of type and dose of oestrogen on the blood pressure of post-menopausal women. Maturitas 1983;5:135.

94. Ziel HK, Finkle WD: Increased risk of endometrial carcinoma among users of conjugated estrogens. N Engl J Med 1975;293:1167.